DESIGN FOR MOVEMENT

DESIGN FOR MOVEMENT

A Textbook on Stage Movement

by

LYN OXENFORD

J. GARNET MILLER LTD : LONDON
THEATRE ARTS BOOKS : NEW YORK

Manufactured in the United States of America

Published in Great Britain by

J. GARNET MILLER, LTD.
129 St. John's Hill
London SW11 1TD, England

ISBN 0-85343-557-X

Published in the United States of America by

THEATRE ARTS BOOKS
153 Waverly Place
New York, New York 10014

ISBN 0-87830-561-0

Second edition
Sixth printing, 1983

Note for American Edition: The reader's attention is called to the fact that in the theatre language of Great Britain the word "producer" refers to the person who in the United States is called a "director". And the British equivalent of the U.S. "producer" is known as a "manager". Since this book was written in England, it was thought wise to leave these terms as they were in the author's manuscript.

THE EDITOR

CONTENTS

PREFACE

THIS book is intended for those amateurs or professionals who, as actors or producers, are interested in stage movement of every kind, but have neither the time nor inclination for a complete training in the various forms of dance. It must be stressed that it is concerned with the use of movement for actors; it is not intended to train dancers. Movement is here used to mean not only the physical transference of the body from place to place, but gestures, mannerisms, positions and grouping.

This has been approached from two angles. First, the psychological, which will be of use to actors and producers of realistic plays, and second, the external, which is intended for actors and producers of stylised plays, pageants, tableaux and religious plays.

The first approach is necessary as so many actors seem unable to form a clear idea of the picture they are presenting to the audience, because of a lack of understanding of the importance of every curve and angle of the body. There seems no happy medium between the fully trained dancer turned actor, and the deliberately under-playing, natural type of actor who performs with little or no attempt at using the body. Amateurs, almost of necessity, fall into the second category. Many Little Theatres have training schools but here again the young members' classes are usually "Expressionistic Movement" where the students express themselves as abstractions—Blue or Flame Groups, or possibly "Revolt". This is, of course, excellent training for the body and the imagination, but it often does not help an inexperienced actor to move effectively in the type of role he is later asked to take in a realistic play. He is probably too much absorbed by his physical effort, during class time, to realise how to relate it to the part of a modern young man. In such exercises there is often no statement as to where the audience is, and very little understanding, on the student's part, of what he is actually meant to be conveying to them. The exercises, in point of fact, are working towards a ballet performance, rather than towards a play with a script. If he is really expressing Flame, which is also on the programme, a script is obviously superfluous.

The first section of this book, therefore, deals with the variety of movement that can and should be used to complement the script, and the particular way of achieving it for the average performer.

The second section of the book deals with the external approach which is successful in beginners' groups, or youth clubs, where group self-consciousness has to be overcome. Puppetry is often the medium chosen to introduce self-conscious people to acting, but the danger of this is that it enables individuals to hide completely, and evade the personal responsibility of facing an audience. The external method provides a mask behind which they can learn and gain self-confidence to appear as actors in their own right.

It is not my object to lay down a hard and fast set of rules of movement, but rather to give students a framework in the two complementary parts of this book, on which they themselves can build with freedom and authority.

LYN OXENFORD

London, August 1951

DESIGN FOR MOVEMENT

PART ONE

THE INDIVIDUAL

CHAPTER I

THE ACTOR'S PATTERN
OF MOVEMENT

LONG ago a famous amateur announced "Gentles perchance you wonder at our show. But wonder on till truth make all things plain"—and that is undoubtedly what some readers of this chapter must keep in mind.

Characterisation of movement and gestures is the great difficulty for so many amateur actors and actresses, and the following way of working out a part has been helpful to those who have tried it. It has proved considerably easier when taught verbally and practically than when written down; hence the quotation at the head of this chapter. The reader is urged to continue undaunted as the Athenian players until all things are plain. Some people understand problems more quickly if explained in one way, others if explained in another, and it is not always possible to write of practical matters in such a way that everyone will easily follow them step by step. Some people are helped by maps and diagrams, others are baffled and bewildered by them. Some find it better to read the entire instructions so that they grasp the general idea, and then recapitulate the details; others must understand each point before going on to the next. This type of mind will possibly find this particular chapter difficult.

Acting must usually convey to the audience something within that audience's comprehension, therefore a compromise often has to be made between what is meant, by the author, to be presented, and what is theatrically effective and possible. The framework here suggested is offered as the result of personal experience of the particular difficulties of amateurs, and has proved of practical use to them.

The particular plan of this book covers a great deal of ground, so the examples, either of exercises, set scenes, or individual business have all been chosen as typical of the average work needed by whatever group is referred to in the context. The plan of alluding to "Mr. George" and "Miss Georgina" instead of "the actor" and "the actress" is used to bring home the fact that the work is for a genuine person, not an impossible ideal. It has been realised that unique problems, highly unusual plays, and abnormal character parts occur in every actor's life, but it has been felt more helpful to concentrate on the average type of performer, in the average type of part, in probably a better than average type of play. Few people care to put a vast amount of time and thought into a badly written part in a flimsy play (although it is in these circumstances that it is mostly needed).

There is often a certain amount of wasted talent among the young members of an amateur company, mainly because they have little or no knowledge of how to plan their work. Great artists do instinctively what lesser folk have to work out the hard way, and the physical characterisation of a part is a perfect example of this.

No one can take short cuts in acting, but an actor must be sure in what direction he is travelling. Characteristic movement springs from *Character*, and the actor must never think of it as an extra, or collect a repertoire of unrelated gestures. This is a waste of time which is badly needed to study the fundamental causes of various types of movements.

It is important and rewarding for actors to observe

people in all their movements, and from these to assess their temperaments and characteristics. From an acting viewpoint, not only understanding of the characters is learnt but simultaneously also how to present them to the audience, e.g. to display to them patterns of movement normally by that character. Even to stand in a position unfamiliar to the actor, but characteristic of the part to be played, is an immense help in creating, in the actor, the mood to be projected to the audience.

Everyone has a *psychological pattern of movement* (i.e. does things in a certain way) which is reflected in his body in a triple rhythm, a Pattern in Space, a Pattern in Time, and a Pattern in Force. This means roughly that one type of person will move in long strides (space), make slow gestures (time) and express himself readily in gesture (force).

The phrase "Pattern in Time" has been used, not as jargon, but because it is very important to understand that each person has a pattern, gestures and movements, that are repeated in the same way that a pattern repeats. *Repetitive patterns* occur not only in types but in individuals, and the triple rhythm should be considered and co-ordinated in all acting movement. Worked out in this way the character will be an integrated person, and hold the audience's attention in a real as well as a theatrical way. When movement is spoken of in this connection, it is taken to include not only the moving of the body from place to place, but all gestures, postures, and mannerisms springing from emotion, character, and circumstance.

Individuals express themselves, whatever the circumstances, in a typically individual form of pattern, e.g., angles, curves, straight lines or diagonal lines. These run very true to form, and are not so much dependent on the physical build of the individual, as on his psychological state. Large people are often extremely neat and economical in their pattern, and small people can pass through a room like a whirlwind leaving destruction in their wake. Therefore, it is impossible to give advice on how the part of a tall man, or a short woman should be played unless their mental make-up is also known. Curving movements will be noticed very often in the bullying type of person, who blusters in order to cover up moral cowardice. This person will invariably go through a crowded street with one shoulder leading, and even in an empty room will use a curved approach to mantelpiece or window.

Diagonal lines will be used by indecisive people who are easily diverted from their original plan of action. These are the people who will stray across the road inviting death from every car, or go upstairs to fetch one article, and come down three hours later having done half a dozen other jobs, but without bringing down the article for which they ascended. The diagonal lines are short, and go in every direction rather like featherstitching, or the veining in a leaf.

Straight lines are usually the sign of a clear thinking controlled person with well-directed energies.

Angles usually mean bad physical co-ordination and an impatience of detail. People who have strong ideas and strong prejudices are to be found in this group. Notably intellectual people very often use this pattern, and those whose minds have a wide grasp of various subjects.

Watch for all the patterns in everyday life and notice how some of them are repeated in every fifth person, and others are very rare and difficult to find.

It is strongly stressed that these are the repetitive patterns, and that emotion can break them. But the mere fact that they are so consistent on ordinary occasions means that the term "pattern" is justified. Mr. George should not mix his pattern on the stage for the perfectly understandable reason that one pattern gesture leaves him in the right control to do another gesture of the same pattern. If he is playing the part of a person with a small neat pattern of time, space and force, and has chosen a small chair for his seat, he cannot justifiably throw himself on the chair from his full height and then suddenly gather in his arms and legs closely without looking like a conjuring trick rather than an actor.

What must be made absolutely clear is that these movements are the reflection of an *habitual* mental attitude, with variations according to the transitory emotions felt. It is possible, however, to consider the *habitual* mental attitude and work out the *habitual* physical attitude, to discover how certain types walk, sit, lie, and carry through the normal matters of their lives. It is still within this pattern that the player must seek to discover how they will move in the abnormal matters of their lives.

The inhibited person will rarely make a violently dramatic gesture whatever the crisis, whereas the uninhibited person who is accustomed to making sweeping gestures will not, in a crisis, make short jerky ones. The second would, if furious, be capable of sweeping everything off the breakfast table, the first would find the same amount of emotional vent in banging the lid on the coffee pot. When studying a character, after deciding on the type of mind he has, and the state of mind in which the play finds him, there is always a difficulty in translating these into the bodily effects that the audience sees. Acting must display, otherwise an audience is unnecessary. In radio the responsibility rests on the voice and the sound engineer.

First, *the pattern in space*. Each person habitually creates his own *acting area*. Let Mr. George take a careful look around the next 'bus in which he travels, and this will be most obvious. People can sit huddled up because they are cold, because they are bewildered, because they have indigestion, because they are afraid of being hit by Gestapo guards if they sit up. It is not always possible to judge which of these reasons applies to any stranger. Mr. George must begin by studying people whose movements are familiar to him and checking up on how often his deductions are right. This need not stop him from observing and remembering the movements and attitudes of strangers, which he can continue to note and docket in his memory for variety of pattern.

Given, theoretically, the same amount of space to sit in, it is instructive to observe the use made of it by five different people, whom we will assume to be under no physical or mental compulsion to sit in any other way than to display their normal pattern.

1. A large fat man, his legs crossed into the gangway, his paper spread full out, blocking the view of the next stop from all behind him.

2. A small woman, baskets on each side of her, leaning forward, her elbow resting on the back of the seat in front of her.

3. A short, thin man, his knees wide apart, his legs stretched, resting on his heels, his hands in his pockets so that his elbow pushes his neighbour practically through the window.

4. A monumental woman, sitting like a massive block, her feet together, her elbows in, her hands clasped on lap, her back erect.

5. An excessively tall, thin man, his feet tucked under his seat, his knees together, his arms folded across his chest.

No one could say these people expressed their physical types in the amount of acting area they use, but they clearly and unmistakable express their mental make-up.

1. An individualist who adjusts himself to unavoidable circumstances (he spreads his legs into the gangway rather than crowd his neighbour), rather unimaginative (as he spreads his paper in front of the view without realising it). He is not purely selfish as he has already considered his neighbour about his legs. He feels the people next to him, therefore he adjusts his legs; he has not sufficient

imagination to visualise the people behind him, therefore he spreads his paper.

2. Taken up by the importance of her own affairs (her baskets have a right to the seat), determined to have her rights, and possessive (the grasp on seat in front which is technically part of her fare).

3. This is a selfish and agressive type who, although he can easily feel he is crowding the other person, does not care. He may have an inferiority complex and be compensating himself in this way.

4. Controlled or lethargic types both sit this way but the controlled type has the erect back.

5. A considerate type anxious to efface himself (his feet tucked under), rather suspicious of any infringement of his personal liberty; he has no desire to have the common touch (arms folded across his chest to preserve immunity, not merely arranged in small space).

These are all real people using real patterns; the actor's job is to select enough of the significant part of the pattern to convince the audience of the reality of what is seen. Unless he maintains it as a pattern the gestures are going to hinder instead of help. The amount of space a person habitually takes up is a valuable clue to his or her habitual mental attitude, so the actor must help the audience by showing them this. The truth of this pattern is at once seen if one applies it to animals. Everyone has, at some time, known when a favourite dog was feeling ill, merely by noticing that it was curled up tightly instead of sprawling as usual. Animals make their patterns very clear to their owners.

It is not proposed here to suggest pattern or lack of pattern for people who suffer from a definite mental illness. It is wiser in such circumstances to consult an expert on the distinctive habits and movements belonging to whatever malady is being portrayed. This may lead to its own difficulty, experts being not yet agreed on the precise

nature of the neurosis from which Hamlet was suffering
or even in which part of the play he was suffering from
any. Dr. Charlotte Woolfe has a most illuminating chapter,
"The Pathology of Gesture", in her book on this subject,
A Psychology of Gesture; it is a textbook well worth con-
sulting in this connection.

The Pattern of Space will be considered first by Mr.
George as it is the easiest pattern to work out, and it is
simplest for him to start by imagining the character in
repose just as he looked at the characters in the 'bus. He
will then make up his mind how the character sits, lies,
and stands habitually.

Repose is such a vitally important thing in acting and
not nearly often enough seen in amateur players. One
reason is that Mr. George has not sufficiently studied the
individual pattern, and therefore directly he ceases to
take active part in the scene, is apt to be left in a pose out
of keeping with the character. Unless a movement is
going to contribute something to the play, it is much
better not to use it; fidgetting, until the right position is
found, takes attention away from what is significant in
the scene. Practical exercises for this section are given
in Chapter V.

The next step is the *pattern in time*: how quickly or
how slowly people usually move. This is a way to judge.
Suppose Mr. George is sitting in a room at home with the
door closed, and someone comes in at the front door and
goes upstairs, he is quite capable of judging which member of the family it is. Even supposing it is 6.30, the time
a particular member always comes in, he would know
immediately if, instead of that person, some stranger
came in and went upstairs, and he would know by the
pace, hurried or slow, of their movements. Long slow
steps, long hasty strides, short stumping steps, short
clicking steps, short padding steps, are all different patterns in time.

How much horror the scene in *Treasure Island* gains by Pew's slowly tapping stick, and how reassured Jim Hawkins would have felt by the sound of the Squire's walking stick, striking quickly on the ground. Pace can be altered by illness, and slowed down considerably, but it will be altered in proportion to the character's habitual pattern. This phase of working out the character helps enormously with the memorising of the lines. Once the pace of the character is established, the rhythm of the sentences helps the rhythm of the gestures, and vice versa. A part which is written with a number of disjointed sentences, dashes and staccato sentences, even though the character is not in an emotional state, needs to be studied most carefully from this point of view. Try to visualise a player arranging flowers on the stage, which is a favourite device of producers. This is an extremely character-revealing business, all too often completely thrown away. Either the player is self-conscious, and is so pleased at being given "something to do with her hands" that she does not bother how she does it, or she is self-conscious in another way and poses prettily. Both actresses display their own characters but not much else.

Whether the scene is tense or relaxed different types would still perform this act differently.

The downright, straightforward and practical character would see to the essentials, enough water, stalks carefully cut, large enough vase, and take her time over this part, rather than the actual arrangement of the blossoms.

An artistic egotistical type would spend the time on an arrangement that was beautiful and drew attention to her talent.

An impatient, arrogant, selfish type would probably ram all the flowers in too tightly, and spend her time mopping up the water which overflowed.

It is clear then that under any violent emotion these types will continue with the same movements, intensified in their individual pattern, rather than change with each other. A sudden slow movement on the part of someone who has up to that moment moved with rapidity and decision, or a brusquely abrupt gesture from an habitually torpid mover can make an enormous impact.

The whole question of making important points is bound up with the pattern in time. "Timing" to so many people means the delivery of a line, or a pause in exactly the right place. Far too few consider it in relation to gesture as just described.

The *pattern in force* concerns the voice rather more than the body, although the body plays its part. This is the pattern which makes one person lay the table with every plate thumped emphatically into place, while another strokes the tablecloth smooth, and slides the glasses along it. It could almost be called a pattern in sound, and that must always be borne in mind.

The direct, honest, unimaginative types habitually use a great deal more force than the imaginative artistic types, who tend to reserve their force for emotional occasions, not to dissipate it on everyday actions. Force is the pattern that is more affected by the emotions than any other, it usually stays within its framework, but may on occasion break out of it. Self-control is a very strong power, and imposes its bonds of restraint and silence, just as much as lack of control will show in wild movement and a loud voice.

These briefly are the three repetitive patterns which have to be co-ordinated if the character is to be fully displayed. Constant observation of real people is the only way to acquire a knowledge of the variety of patterns possible, but the student will very quickly notice the repetitive gestures and link them up with mental outlook. Equally he will see cliché gestures in real life that, while perfectly genuine, would not carry conviction on any stage.

The types mentioned here are straightforward and easily classified as far as their patterns and bodily display are concerned. Much of the subtlety of interpretation will probably come from the voice with which this book does not deal in any way. In many a crisis in the play Mr. George will have to convey his thoughts and emotions through his voice, while standing perfectly still. So it is essential that he shall know how to stand, so that the audience will not be distracted from what he is saying. When he has understood the mental make-up of the character that he has been chosen to play, and worked out the corresponding physical pattern that he intends to use, he can advance, hand in hand with Miss Georgina, who has kept pace with him in her own work, into the next chapter. Here they will begin to cope practically with the fusion of their own ideas of their parts, and their personal equipment for carrying them out theatrically.

CHAPTER II

THE CHARACTER DISPLAYED

THERE is a great deal of interest in what is known as the "Stanislavsky Method" in the amateur theatre, and this is all to the good, except when it tends to become bogus and pretentious posing. There is a feeling that, because Mr. George knows instinctively (but not from the script) that the character has a cross-eyed cousin in Constantinople who does bead embroidery on Thursday and eats carraway seeds, he has done all his preliminary work. Sometimes there is tendency to go so far behind the script that he might as well not go on the stage at all, for all the attention he can spare to acting, and a lofty disregard of the audience, to the extent of not using his body to convey anything. It is always much easier to imagine beautiful and dramatic methods of playing characters, than to buckle down to the hard work of presenting them. As long as it is all in his own mind, no one can criticise or contradict him. It is the ghastly moment when the pro ducer says, "No, no, that means absolutely nothing when you do it that way; what on earth are you trying to convey?", that Mr. George feels the need for bodily technique to carry out his ideas. So he must *plot the part physically*.

Movements, mannerisms, gestures: he knows what the character does, he knows what it thinks, but his own body is definitely not the same as that of the character, and he does not know how to bridge the gap. He thinks of a mannerism, tapping his thumb with his pince-nez, and then he thinks of another, perhaps looking at an old-fashioned watch, snapping it open and shut. The two mannerisms are used incessantly throughout the play, "to establish character". They are probably not used when they would be most effective, to point a plot line or mark a pause; they are just used as mannerisms in a void.

Mr. George has not co-ordinated his mental picture and his physical body, mainly because he has not realised the acting possibilities of his whole body. What he needs is to be shown how to work out for himself a *framework* of movement for the type of character, and how he can use that framework within the framework of the play, and build up *detail*. When he has done this, his energy can be devoted to presenting the results to the audience, with the satisfying feeling that all his previous mental work on the character will now be appreciated, because it is couched in a theatrically effective way.

The framework should begin with a clear mental picture of two things. Firstly, the physical and psychological type of the character to be played, which governs the gestures, movements, and mannerisms he will habitually use, quite apart from any emotional scenes.

Secondly, the physical type of Mr. George himself, and exactly how it differs from the character. Having worked this out he can then go on to decide which habitual gestures of his own he must entirely eliminate, which he can modify to fit the character, and which habitual gestures of the character he will select to use in the scenes of dramatic and emotional power. The average performer does not work in this way, for one so often sees a carefully imagined character, betrayed at a vital moment by a movement which is ludicrously inadequate and out of place.

The usual way seems to be a suggestion from the actor or producer that a certain movement should be made. Reading the script (and carrying out what he thinks Stanislavsky meant) Mr. George beats on the table. "No, no", says the producer, "that is quite out of character— try something else."

"Like this", says Mr. George hopefully, beating twice instead of four times.

"No, something quite different", says the producer, coping simultaneously with a cat walking about the stage, the caretaker hissing that they must be out of the hall by 9.30, and a worried stage manager asking if they shall have canteen now or wait for a few minutes.

"Like this," says Mr. George magnanimously, thumping the table once instead of twice.

"No, no, we will have to think of something else, carry on for now", says the producer. Mr. George, feeling that he had produced no less than three different ideas, and still not been satisfactory, probably decides to let the producer suggest something next time. Next time, they start the play just after this scene; the time after that, canteen arrives at the critical moment, and eventually it is tacitly accepted by both that he makes a vague thumping noise, and honour is satisfied.

The quality of active *co-operation by the actors* for the good of the play, quite apart from any personal success they may make in their parts, is what so often marks the difference between the professional attitude of mind in the theatre from that of the amateur. The amateur actor is all too often sincere in his desire for the good of the play, but he is passive in his co-operation with the producer and fellow actors, diffident, although painstaking, in his ideas about his part, bringing up the rear rather than blazing the trail.

The excuse is often given that there was not enough time for rehearsals. If each actor in the case spent each journey to and from work each day thinking exclusively about the part he was playing, developing technically its possibilities of intonation and variety of speed, imagining the exact number of steps he had to take for each move, precisely where and how he was standing to take each cue, where he wanted to get laughs, and where, and how long he could pause and still keep the audience's attention;

not only would he have much more fun, but rehearsals would achieve far more.

So often, at amateur rehearsals the producer has to work desperately hard to clear the ground each time because with the lapse of days between rehearsals, the actors have not acquired the habit of thought about their part. Producers usually live with their productions, otherwise they do not take on the job, but the actors and actresses tend towards a wheelbarrow state of mind in which they are competent when pushed and told where to go, but, when the impetus is removed, are unable to carry on under their own steam.

The producer can always be trusted to stop overplaying, and it is a comparatively simple thing to scale it down, but the producer has many things to watch besides the playing of one person. The actor's responsibility is heavy within its own limits, and it goes far beyond just following the producer's instructions.

The average actor finds it very difficult to visualise himself, and to see that a crossed leg or a hand in the pocket can contribute to the other actor's playing as well as his own. For instance, two men are sitting one each side of a small table, one talking, one listening—the listener is sitting slightly sideways to the table, leaning his left elbow on it with the hand on the table, his other hand in his trouser pocket, his legs crossed. At a given moment in the other's speech a plot point must be put across or the attention of the audience must be sharpened. The listener, by abruptly moving his right hand to grasp the top of his chair, thus thrusting his right shoulder forward, will create more tension and urgency. The right shoulder shuts off the other people and encloses the two of them in a more intimate grouping. Yet again and again, when rehearsing a gesture of this type, one finds the actor just has a general impression that he moved, and finds it extraordinarily difficult to recapture the exact attitude just described.

There was a scene in the play *There shall be no Night* in which Alfred Lunt, the American actor, playing the part of the Father, overheard the news of his son's death. Mr. Lunt was standing by the window with his back to the audience, stiff with horror and grief. As a full realisation of his loss came over him one could see the rigid effort to control it, all through his tense body, for a few seconds. Then the agony was too much for him, and it *leaked* out through one heel, which ground into the carpet.

There are several lessons to be learnt from this. It is not supposed for one moment that Mr. Lunt thought to himself what was the most unusual way to express grief, and decided on his heel· It is suggested that Mr. Lunt, while thoroughly realising that character's feelings, also used a consummate technique to express it. Cliché gestures of grief cease, after a time, to have an effect on the audience; but many people saw that gesture, they all remembered it and commented on how strong a feeling of grief came across the footlights. Such is Mr. Lunt's talent for projection, that there is no doubt at all he could equally well have stood quite still and raised tears, but the significant fact is that he, even he, did use a gesture to help the audience.

The second lesson is, that sometimes when an amateur does work out something like this, and finds he is unavoidably standing behind a small table, it will be unseen. Perhaps he asks if the table can be moved, and it is then found that it cannot be, because later on in the play a letter has to be put on it to be picked up by another actor. From this point the situation diverges sharply between amateur and professional. The amateur sees reason, gives up his cherished gesture, and relies on pure projection. The professional will fight to retain what he feels is important to his conception of the part. He will ask if the letter can be put on the sideboard instead. The actor who has to pick up the letter will then co-operate, probably suggesting that the table is moved nearer the centre to clear this gesture, or if he pauses on his entrance, he can take two steps less and reach it on the same cue. If this is not practical, the actor works out something else which will be above table level, and still express what he wants, possibly even using the table as a help. This co-operation between actors is most important.

The time for trying things out is not always at rehearsal, but sometimes at home in front of a mirror. The drawback to this is that, naturally, as the head turns to look, part of the pose goes. It is an interesting experiment to take up a stylised or period attitude facing the mirror with the eyes closed, then to open them, and to check on the difference between imagination and fact. In most cases what feels like, and is intended to be, an arm outstretched in a gracious curve, is nothing of the sort. The arm sags at the elbow, finishes with a drooping wrist and crooked little finger, and looks neither decorative nor dramatic, and not even real. An elbow flung up in front of the face conveys something quite different from a hand flung in front of the face, and yet nine out of ten will merely make a note of "arm gesture". Whether to raise one shoulder, or both, is a question that rarely occurs to people, it is just a shrug; but let them do it in front of a mirror, and they will immediately see the importance of the choice. One of the most dramatic gestures in history was achieved with the utmost economy of effort, the turned down thumb of the Roman Emperor when the gladiator had to die.

Many actors can feel the character completely before they even enter, but are incapable of opening the door easily. It is necessary to realise that gestures and everyday movements have on occasion to be unobtrusive, although they need never be uncharacterised.

Practise the following exercise and time it with a stop-watch to see how quickly it can be done without the effect of haste.

Start with hat, coat and loose gloves on. Put right hand round left knuckles and draw left glove off, still holding it in the right hand. Put left hand round right knuckles and draw off right glove with left glove, and put both into left hand pocket. Grasp coat in centre of collar back with left hand travelling from left pocket, and pull it off, guiding with right hand until it can hang over left arm. Raise both hands to hat, if it is tight, lifting from each side so as not to disarrange hair, take hat off and hold in left hand. This method takes a long time to write, but it is economical in time and space, and most unobtrusive. It avoids taking up space by the waving of the coat over the head like a lassoo while struggling to get out of it arm by arm, which is the snare for the inexperienced.

It is valuable practice to work out other usual actions, such as opening doors, pouring out wine, etc., and then eliminate every unnecessary flourish, and it is always a good plan to work with a stop watch and check progress. Needless to say, there must be no cheating in pace, the same speed must be maintained each time, the time saved must count either in the actions being done more quickly, or in the elimination of certain gestures in order to make time for emphasis. These actions can also be practised, still entirely without emotion, as an old person or an invalid would do them, slowly and with difficulty.

An example of a slow exercise is to take off gloves very slowly, pulling each finger off separately, blow into them, smooth them out, and fold them out carefully. To do this slowly but continuously, never actually pausing, needs careful control. For timing with speech, or pointing a speech, try saying the alphabet and finishing accurately on Z. Then try it emphasising each vowel sound on a definite finger (A on the thumb, E on the fourth finger for instance). Then do it as rapidly as possible, counting as rapidly as possible, for co-ordination of movement and speech; and finally work it into any long speech of any suitable play, until it is possible to gauge exactly how long such an action, done at any given speed should take. Egg timers can be most useful where exact timing of gesture is concerned.

An inexperienced player will often find his greatest difficulty lies in simply having to cross from one side of the stage to the other, because walking is something usually taken for granted, and therefore he does not know how to analyse it. The first thing to remember is that stage illusion usually demands, no matter how small the actual space available, that it should appear not to cramp the actors. When a cross could be made with two strides, it is advisable to take five smaller steps; when a character apparently rushes madly across the stage, it must not actually be a head-long run, but a carefully counted and poised progression.

The weight should be so balanced that it can easily be transferred from one foot to the other, and as a general rule the move starts with the free foot; it is better not to give a little shuffle, but make a clear-cut step. If the down-stage foot is forward and a turn has to be made, either turn up-stage leaving the feet in their open up-stage position, or bring the up-stage foot forward and turn down-stage, still with the feet in an open position. Practise the following movements until they can be done easily and unconsciously with no worry about balance or timing, leaving the mind and emotions free to concentrate on the acting of the role:

Walking forwards and backwards and turning.
Running forwards and backwards and turning.
Running forwards looking backwards and turning.
Running forwards looking forwards.
Running forwards, sudden halt, walking slowly backwards.
Walking backwards, pausing, turning, and running forward.

Walking across a stage briskly, pausing as if struck by a sudden thought, turning and retracing steps slowly.

The last is a particularly useful exercise as it involves judging the distance so that when the pause comes, the proper foot is forward for the turn, and when the steps have been retraced the last step finishes on the correct foot. This should be repeated in varying areas until the eye is trained to measure space and calculate how many steps are needed to fit it. Nothing looks worse than a player taking two enormous strides and then marking time on the same spot until the cue comes for him to return. The main secret of controlled movement of this type is relaxed knees, and a step that starts with a stretch from the thigh. If the knees are relaxed, the heel, when walking, and the ball of the foot, when running, can be placed on the ground in a controlled way and exactly where they are intended to go; there will be no skidding or crashing. If the leg is stretched from the thigh, not from the knee, it will help to give the illusion that the actor is not cramped by space, it shows a better line to the audience, and is easier to control or retract if the distance is miscalculated.

Sitting down is another simple action that is often made unnecessarily obtrusive. The distance to the seat should be measured by the eye, and the number of steps calculated so that the last step is neither a slide to reach the chair, nor does it continue until the chair acts as a buffer and forcibly stops the move.

The possibilities of variety of position while sitting are sadly underrated both by Miss Georgina and Mr. George. Both tend to adopt a lady-like position facing either dead front or dead profile, which they maintain fixedly until an actual move has to be made; with legs crossed and hands in pockets (Mr. George), or clutching handbag (Miss Georgina).

Let us take first the chair, and then the bodies, and debate what can de done with them.

The actor can sit on the seat, the back, or on either of the arms; the chair can be turned round and straddled with ease, or, if it is solid enough, the player can sit on the back, resting his feet on the seat. The players can sit with bodies sideways on the seat, can lie at full length with their legs out-stretched and their arms behind their heads. They can sit forward, their elbows resting on wide-spread knees, chin on hands, or their hands clasped between knees. They can sit on the edge of the seat with feet twined round the legs or the rungs of the chair and hands clasped round elbows. They can sit sideways on the seat with backs turned towards audience, head over shoulder, hands clasping back of chair, or still sideways on seat, one elbow resting on back of chair, hand resting against head, the other hand sustaining the balance by holding on the other side or arm of the chair. They can even (if the producer sees fit) move the chair a fraction nearer to any other article of furniture and put their feet up. They can stand on the chair for a moment of excitement, or fling it over for a moment of temper. Whether the legs are crossed at the ankles or the knees; or whether one leg is crossed over the other, the crossed ankle resting on the other knee; or whether the legs are crossed tailor fashion so that the position is compact on the seat of the chair; their attitudes all add up to more interesting patterns for the audience to watch.

For Miss Georgina a feminine and yearning position can be assumed by sitting on the chair facing front, then throwing the weight on hip to turn slightly towards the hero, and resting the same elbow on the back of the chair. This gives considerable range of movement so that she can yearn either more towards him, or less, as the dialogue demands. All through these positions it must be clearly comprehended when sideways to the audience, or sideways on the seat of the chair is intended. Many more things can be worked out once the players start thinking along these lines to carry out their own ideas and those of the producer.

They must always remember and consider the audience and cultivate an affection for it—it will respond by noticing good work, appreciating detail and giving them support and comfort in difficult scenes.

The most expert technical work may fail to hold an audience and be effort wasted. To weave the thread of emotion that crosses the footlights and binds both sides together is the actor's ultimate aim, and the knowledge that this has been achieved is his reward. Audiences can be bullied or they can be coaxed, but they must never be ignored by either Miss Georgina or Mr. George. The art of acting should be an unselfish one, and consideration for their fellow actors and the audience a matter of course.

CHAPTER III

OVERTONES AND INFLUENCES

THE personal patterns of individuals reflecting their mental make-up have already been dealt with, but there are also the overtones made by environment, race and heredity. In plays the characters often appear in their own environment which is comparatively straightforward, but should they be shipwrecked, let us say, then the actors must use their own imagination to build up their past surroundings. Racial influences fluctuate according to how long the person has been in a foreign country, and Mr. George should read this section completely and carefully, otherwise he will leap to wrong conclusions. He must notice to which group the character belongs— artists, artisans, socialites or intellectuals, as well as to which group of countries he belongs. Psychologically the same types recur, but environment plays a large part in how they behave outwardly.

Consider the movements of a person whose daily *occupation* makes heavy physical demands. The normal resting attitude would be one that relaxed the muscles used in work; for instance a ballet dancer would relax completely by lying flat on a sofa or in a hammock, or on the floor, as every muscle is used; a washer woman usually would fold her arms across her stomach and rest her shoulders.

The vocational type of work, nurse, nun, dancer, which is deliberately chosen as a way of life, not merely a job, ties up with the psychological side rather than the physical. A nurse or nun will normally stand in a controlled position not only because she has been trained to stand quietly, but because her whole attitude of mind has to be controlled.

An interesting point is that people with a markedly scientific mind often find it extremely difficult to move in time to music. They keep their own rhythm and refuse to have any other imposed on them. As a general rule it has been found that people who cannot move in time to music are in psychological stress, and people who cannot balance easily are inhibited. This was proved often in the black-out, which the extroverts found far easier to cope with than the introverts. Physical balance is very largely a question of self-confidence and trust in the outside world, and when lacking is a most difficult thing to correct. It must be tackled mentally.

There is the familiar situation of the acrobat, jealous of his wife, failing at the critical moment of balance, and being quite literally upset. It would be useless for an actor to play the part of an acrobat if his own balance roused doubts in the audience's mind. One sees a business secretary on the stage (referred to as "My right hand for fifteen years") bungle while putting a sheet of paper in her typewriter. This actress had not grasped the fact that even an unvocational job imposes a physical habit. Such a person would do this act mechanically and use, unconsciously, the most economical method of getting the work done. This refers not to every typist, but to the character just described. Even slipshod and careless people develop, in their daily work, an economy of gesture that they do not use in their private life. To portray any character with a profession or job, it is as well to remember this continually.

When the job or profession demands any sort of special costume, the gestures made at work will tend to appear in private life, even when that costume is not being worn. Someone accustomed to wearing an academic gown, with its backward drag will make the same hitching gesture to adjust its weight, even when wearing a tweed jacket which fits on the shoulders. People who wear glasses at work, will put up a hand to adjust them even when they are not wearing them. A nurse will automatically smooth her cuffs at the wrist when she is in fact wearing a short sleeved dress, and a housewife used to wearing an apron, will catch herself wiping her hands on her best frock. Farmers' gaiters, policemen's helmets, soldiers' uniforms, all tend to restrain movement, and will help to suggest mannerisms.

The use of costume in gesture is most helpful, but should never degenerate into fidgetting. An example of effective movement was seen in *Man about the House*. Two women were sitting on a sofa chatting about Italy. One had a line, "Oh! I adore colour", and on the last word she suddenly unfolded a fan, which had been lying unnoticed on her lap, into a sweep of cerise feathers. The whole audience sat up and gasped. Had she been restlessly waving the fan previously, the effect would have been lost; it was the intelligently sudden use of it that made the point.

Mannequins learn how to show off the best points of a dress, playing with a scarf to draw attention to it. It is reasonable to suppose that a mannequin in private life would automatically adjust herself to the most becoming attitude in whatever she was wearing.

An exercise on this for the student is to take a classified Trade Directory, and see how many trades he knows, or can imagine, from the point of view of occupational gestures and relaxed positions. Common sense will rule out trifling distinctions; sedentary factory workers, whether making buttons or boxes, would probably need the same relaxing movements, although anyone employed in making something will be interested in picking up and examining that object when it it seen elsewhere.

Racial patterns are varied and fall into categories of groups of countries rather than individual countries. These groups are, roughly, the Latin countries, the Scandinavian, the Teutonic, the Anglo-Saxon, and the American. They are very much bound up with the different upbringing and language used in the different countries.

Class consciousness has a definite influence in the categories. Generally speaking, all the highly educated members of all the groups of countries will be more self-controlled and restrained than the uneducated. The middle classes will steer a middle course, and artists and intellectuals have always been universal in their habits and easily charted in any country.

Aristocrats from these groups of countries would have more similarity with each other in their style of gesture than they would with a labourer in their own country. Royal Courts, even though now steadily disappearing, have held sway so long that they have formed an international code of manners, varying from country to country it is true, but clearly recognisable as etiquette and distinct from behaviour. Allowance must be made for this and the character's background and environment must be understood.

English can be spoken with such a stiff upper lip that the facial muscles need not be disturbed, and English upbringing suppresses the display of emotion, so the average English person controls his gestures, except those done with the feet. Figures of eight drawn on the ground, feet twined round the legs of chairs, feet turned completely out, or turned doggedly in, and feet swinging from toe to heel, can all be constantly observed in an English crowd with unmoved faces and passive hands. Sometimes the impression is given that English people think themselves invisible below the knees, so often do they allow their agitation to be expressed only by their feet.

Americans, possibly as the result of gum chewing, have extraordinarily mobile faces, which they move incessantly. The average American advertisement looks to an English eye as if it exaggerated the facial expression, but this is not so. American mouths are particularly expressive, and can be twisted with extreme dexterity to convey almost any shade of meaning. In a continent so large, many exceptions must be expected, and other things vary from State to State, but this expressive mouth is noticeable everywhere.

Male Americans use a wide pattern in space when in repose. Although arm gestures are not often used to express emotion, the arms and legs are constantly flung full out when either a sitting, standing, or reclining position is taken. The most typical head position is the head shrugged into the shoulders with fore-shortened neck. They adopt a much wider range of body angles than Europeans although their range of gestures is limited. American women are consciously elegant in their pattern, and use a variety of hand and wrist gestures; the typical attitude of the head is a provocative tilt. The average attitude is one of exceeding self-confidence and self-control, but not inhibited: good balance and poise, a strong pattern of force, and a definite pace, either markedly quick, or deliberately slow.

The Latin races share a bodily grace and ease, fluid movements and a sense of rhythm, particularly when natives of the warmer Southern provinces. In the Northern races all these qualities are still inherent, but more controlled and guarded. They have wide range of head movements, exact shoulder and hand gestures, and free arm and waist movement. The pattern in time is quicker than in England, and the pattern in space larger. Most Latins walk as if they could dance well, and have little difficulty in dropping on one knee in a situation which an Englishman would consider only required a handshake. There is a spring and elasticity about their movements that must be noticed, and an elegance in finishing off each little sequence of actions performed. A febrile pattern of force is prevalent. Teutonic races have a slower pattern in time, a heavier force, but not a large space pattern. Shoulder, head and arms move more readily, but more ponderously than in England, and a gesture when made is often held for a considerable time or repeated slowly. They usually sit compactly and walk steadily, with sure direction. Hand gestures are made with a flat palm and straight fingers rather than the Latin curved palm and expressively flickering fingers. A typical head position is that of head slightly on one side, with the chin drawn in or thrust out, making a definite angle in either case. The Scandinavian races appear to be a blend of the two types of contrasting movement. The walk is much lighter and freer than a Teuton, but not so rapid and springy as a Latin. The arm movements are easy and flexible, the hand movements decided and strongly characterised. Strong, erect carriage of head and body, supple waist and hip movements, and an abandonment of unnecessary restriction of physical movement are also characteristic. The pattern of space needs width, depth and height, and is used to its full extent. The pattern in time gives staccato bursts of violent energy, followed by periods of complete lassitude and relaxation. It is most apparent on watching a crowd of Scandinavians how much play is made by the side of the body. The movement forward of one foot will carry with it hip and shoulder in one loose swing, which is exactly repeated as the other foot comes forward. It makes the same pattern in bodies that is seen in the kilts of Highland soldiers swinging past, marching. It does not seem real, so perfectly is it co-ordinated and so effortlessly.

When watching crowds in foreign countries, their racial patterns stand out clearly. Mob emotion is the same everywhere, illogical and infectious, but the way in which it is demonstrated differs sharply from country to country. It differs even in sound, but that is outside this framework, although dialect and accent are so closely tied up with the patterns both of pace and force. If a moving film were shown from the silent film days of a genuine crowd in an excited state, it ought to be possible to say to which of the aforementioned groups it belonged. No attempt is made here to group the Asiatic races as the author knows very little about them and has not had the chance to study them.

The Jewish people are international and retain their own characteristics no matter where they happen to be born. They normally need a rapid tempo, a medium pattern of space, and a nervously exaggerated pattern in force.

Hereditary mannerisms are largely a question of the child copying the parent it admires. In the case of mother and daughter in a play, such mannerisms would give an air of authenticity to the relationship. They would have to be carefully worked out, in character, and not too bizarre. They would defeat their own ends if the audience were at once to start saying to one another, "Look how clever they are, using the same mannerisms"—such things must be kept subtle. It can be either a small gesture, the straightening of a vase each time they pass it, or an emotional gesture at a crisis, grinding one hand into the palm of the other. In the case of father and son it may be a particular stance: legs straddled and head thrust dogmatically forward.

Several play plots have hinged on a gesture betraying the hereditary relationship of two people who are supposed to be strangers, but it is rare to see the idea utilised by actors where it has not been stressed.

Individual handicaps can be physical or mental: too short legs or a lack of rhythm. Physical handicaps should be tackled in two ways: correction and camouflage. Correction can be done by exercises, camouflage by make-up and costume; in both cases the fact that an active effort is being made will help self-confidence.

Exercises are slow but sure if, and only if, they are done

regularly. It is absolutely wasted effort to do them furiously one week and not at all the next, but it is quite miraculous what can be achieved by steady persistence.

There are certain handicaps that are impossible to overcome, and it is better to decide whether to capitalise on them or give up the part. An actor with a shrunken face and short thin legs will never be able to pad himself convincingly for Henry VIII, an actress who is majestic and strongly featured is wiser not to attempt Peter Pan. The radio will give these people all the scope they need, if the parts are outside their physical range but within their vocal and mental ability.

If it is found that certain mannerisms have developed in the player and are being carried on from part to part, the best correction is to ask a friend to make some unobtrusive signal each time the fault occurs, starting from the first rehearsal. This is a thing which is impossible to correct by oneself, but it is also a habit to be nipped in the bud instantly it appears.

Gloves can be used either to draw attention to lovely hand movements, or to conceal ugly or inexpressive ones, while exercises are remedying the faults. A wooden-looking hand, encased in heavy fur mitts, has the same force as a supple, expressive hand similarly enclosed, a point not always realised. A frivolous hat can show off the graceful carriage of a head, and show up the ungainly one.

Mr. George and Miss Georgina must face their faults squarely, and use every possible means to prevent the audience from doing the same thing. Any handicaps for stage work are usually also handicaps in real life, so there is a double incentive to eliminate them. As time is always limited, it is wise to weight up the amount available, and the way it is intended to divide it between developing assets and getting rid of liabilities. Personal feelings are not a good guide on this point; most small dark people would prefer to be tall and fair, and many majestic types long to be kittenish.

Producers are generally good judges of players' assets, and potentialities, and will advise as to whether voice production is the vital need, or whether "the voice beautiful" is ruining every characterisation attempted, as it peals out mellow tones to which its owner listens entranced. From the moment the first role is acted, the player must attempt to judge how far he has achieved what he set out to do, and must not depend entirely on outside criticism. Self judgement in acting is extremely difficult to acquire and some famous professionals have failed to do so. Unless the circumstances are exceptional, an entire audience's reactions are a better guide than any single member of it, as to how far an actor has succeeded in his part. Stage history shows many examples of famous players who have triumphed over physical handicaps—Irving, with his curious voice and movements, Bernhardt, with one leg gone, Esmond Knight, over his blindness—therefore too much stress must not be laid on physical handicaps if they are off-set by qualities of another nature. Imagination, will power, perseverance, insight into character, can all be developed and will all be needed for a convincing performance, whether amateur or professional.

Physical beauty alone can achieve nothing in acting— a comforting thought to those who do not possess it.

CHAPTER IV

PERIOD AND STYLISED MOVEMENT

INEXPERIENCED performers are apt to forget that once they are in front of an audience any garment is "costume", and that the correct handling of a cigarette case is just as important as the correct handling of a crinoline. The attitude of mind, that of being familiar with the clothes, is most important to preserve when wearing garments of any other period. To familiarise themselves with every detail of the costume, how to put it on and take it off, is the first step to being able to exploit its possibilities in gesture and action. Sometimes they feel the character would not have chosen that particular costume, in which case they must visualise the relative who sent it, and who must not be offended by their refusal to wear it. They should know enough of the character to know whether it would be worn, as sent or whether it would be altered to the personal taste.

Period movement, meaning movement in any other than contemporary clothes, is mainly a question of common sense. Three things decide the poise and balance: what is worn on the head, what is worn on the feet, and whether or not corsets are in fashion.

To save time in dealing with this subject I have grouped the movements in a common-sense rather than a chrono logical way. If the costume has heelless shoes, whether they are Grecian sandals, or mediaeval slippers, or Early Victorian dancing shoes, the movement of the foot will be the same. The walk may differ, but it includes the whole body so that must be correlated with the rest of the costume.

Period manners are a most complicated affair, and it is best to consult one of the experts listed in Appendix I for any special period. This is particularly important for amateurs when entering a Festival, as adjudicators generally check up thoroughly beforehand, when confronted with an historical play.

In all ages, most people have cared about both their appearance and their comfort, and it is advisable to bear this in mind whenever in doubt as to how to tackle an unruly costume.

For a young man of to-day, in flannel trousers, wrinkled woollen socks, a high-necked pullover and flopping hair, a comfortable attitude is to lounge in an armchair, probably with one leg over the arm. To a beau of the eighteenth century it would be not only painful but expensive. His silk stockings would ladder, his corsets would cut him, his breeches would split, his cravat would work out, and his wig be pushed awry. In order to be comfortable, he would have to take up an attitude that would seem stiff and uneasy to a modern youth.

In considering costume of any period, it is best to start with the feet. Walking barefoot, or in sandals, is usually easier for men than for women. The walk should be natural, i.e. heel first, then ball, with knees relaxed. It should be realised that the body must be well drawn up if a dignified posture is needed, to counteract the lack of height given by heels. Women dressed in the Jane Austen period, early 1800, often have difficulty walking in the light dancing sandals. They either turn up their toes, or run everywhere on their toes. It is easier to run, but it should not be difficult to walk naturally if small steps are taken. If all the females in the play run everywhere, the correct atmosphere of lady-like control is lost.

Medium heels are comfortable for both sexes and need no further comment. High heels are naturally much easier for women than men. Women have only to be careful that

D

the heels are not too high, as then a bent-kneed gait has to be assumed that is most unsightly on the stage. Men, when putting on high heels for the first time, should take in a deep breath and settle their weight back as they let it out. For men to move with high heels with the right air, needs care and thought about balance, but it is well worth it. Riding boots, jack boots, thigh boots, all dictate their own movements. They are meant for striding, for being hit with a riding whip, for kicking hapless victims, for sitting straddling a chair. No man should have difficulty in wearing them, and they lend themselves admirably to a swashbuckling manner of movement.

Corsets or stiffened bodices are often a bugbear to both sexes. Much the best way to tackle movement in these is to hold the body so that it is as comfortable as possible. Hang up the dress or corset and look at it well to see exactly how it ought to set. Then put it on carefully, draw a deep breath, and find out where there is room for the ribs, where it cramps the body, and where it really fits. Then draw another deep breath, rise on the toes and settle well into the spaces left. Sometimes the weight has to be pushed forward, sometimes tilted back, the bust lifted well away from the waist, or the back more arched than formerly. Stand in the costume until it is familiar, then walk and sit. If it digs sharply into the ribs the posture is not erect enough.

When one considers the occupations available to "Ladies" in Victoria's reign, and reads Florence Nightingale's description of days spent doing useless embroidery, it is hardly surprising that they had plenty of energy to sit erect, and that there was little tired slouching. This leaves out of account the fact that there were corset bones, bodice bones, and crinolines to dig into the body unless an erect position was maintained. The "Madame Recamier Reclining" position, when thin muslin dresses were worn, was a short respite, but corsets soon resumed their hold. It is not usually possible to get the correct corsets for the period, but pictures must be studied if the line is to be held. To look as if one always wore a bustle and carried a parasol, when the costume only arrived for the dress rehearsal is difficult, but must be done.

It is sometimes forgotten that people in past ages were only human, and not at all anxious to wear clothes that they could not move in more or less easily. It may not be possible for moderns to feel as free as in their own clothes, but it should be possible for them to act as freely.

Head-dresses and wigs are the third item with which to reckon. These need to be firmly secured and properly balanced. Each type of head-dress limits the action of the head, but only slightly.

The mediaeval head-dresses for women are rather heavy with a backwards pull. This is balanced by the high waist line, the position of gathering up the skirt in front, as well as by heelless shoes.

Men wearing Charles II costume, complete with ruffles, periwig and feathered hat, will find the long cane a great help in walking and presenting a well-balanced picture.

It must be remembered for how many centuries swordsmanship was part of a man's training. Any duelling or use of the sword in salute must be done expertly, in order to look convincing. To see someone making three or four false attempts to replace his sword in his scabbard is a sorry sight. Duels should be carefully rehearsed, so that they can be played with that enjoyment at practising his skill that a man would naturally feel. It is not always realised what strong fingers and wrists, and excellent footwork are needed for real fencing. If a duel occurs in a later scene in the play, the duellist must give a feeling of strength early on. If he is meant to win the duel, he must not make clumsy or fumbling moves with slack fingers, and then expect the audience to believe in him as an expert swordsman. There is such swift co-ordination between hand and eye in fencing, that it is impossible for clumsy person to become expert at it.

In most historical plays it does not matter if a woman looks inexpert at any form of physical exertion. It is only in the present century that woman has been expected to excel at games. In other centuries, however, she was supposed to know all about housekeeping; therefore any form of spinning, embroidery (however weird the frame) knitting, tatting, crochet, or needlework should be done tidily and efficiently.

Falcons, archery equipment, croquet mallets, need merely be used as attractive accessories. There is no necessity, unless the script refers to it, to pretend to any skill or even knowledge of the sport. Knowledge of the character will help to decide whether a woman would be carrying a bow if she did not intend to compete.

There is such a fascinating range of *hand properties* for the costumes of all periods, that it is illuminating to discover which is the individual choice of the character played. Through the centuries certain types have had certain things: tear bottles, oranges studded with cloves, smelling salts, aspirin bottles for the fastidious people; mirrors, cosmetics, beauty patches, fans, nail varnishes for the beauty seekers; pipes, dog whips, fishing tackle for the masculine men; embroidered gloves, lace handkerchiefs, quizzing glasses for the fashionable men. The handling of these things, in a visually decorative as well as a characteristic way, is a most rewarding study.

It must not be forgotten that in the seventeenth, eighteenth and nineteenth centuries, the teaching of dancing and deportment was done by ballet masters. Ballet positions of the feet, ballet training in the carriage of the head and arms, all help immensely in the portrayal of characters in these periods. Before organised games in girls' schools, the entire stress of physical training (which was never neglected) was on correct posture and deportment. It gave, in a way difficult to visualise nowadays, an immediate sign of social status. "An elegant bearing" was neither expected or encouraged in the lower classes.

Certain qualities were prized in women in some periods, different ones were more valued in others. In some periods certain qualities were accentuated in women's dress and attitude, although in all periods the emphasis oas been on the decorative aspect, when women were presented on the stage. The pendulum has swung regularly between decorum and licence, both in manners and movement. From Saxon to Elizabethan times women moved and sat with dignity and decorum. The clothes looked voluminous and sweeping, but it must not be forgotten that the materials were pure wool and silk, and were not heavy. The head-dress demanded that the head should be well poised, and strong corsets held the waist firmly. From Elizabeth to Cromwell the movement was more sprightly. The farthingale allowed a bouncing walk that was very provocative. The head-dress had dwindled first to a light and becoming coronet, and then to a lace cap, worn at home, and jewels or flowers for ceremonious occasions. The head could, therefore, be tossed and moved with much greater freedom than in the previous era. In Cromwell's time the force of public opinion was so strong as to compel modest behaviour and quiet movement. At the Restoration Court (not in the country districts) wantonness was the mode. The dresses were designed to slip negligently off white shoulders, the curls escaped from their ribbons as the head was thrown back flirtatiously, and bracelets jingled and lace ruffles swayed as the fans moved to and fro. In a Charles II dress, the most typical attitude of the period was to sit half turned sideways on a chair, one arm stretched along the back of it, the other hand on the other arm of the chair, the back slightly arched, head tilted and skirt tastefully disposed in silken folds all around. Court ladies, of whom many portraits exist, were invariably leaning well forward, or well back-ward, with not very much covering on their top halves, and yards and yards of material round their feet. Very, very feminine and seductive were they, with apparently nothing on their minds except the duty to be beautiful.

A short period of formality followed with William III's Court, but from Queen Anne until Victoria, the poses were as coquettish and alluring as the exigencies of their costumes allowed.

The typical stage curtsey, sinking completely to the ground with the back bowed forward so that the head rested practically on the knee, was never used in ordinary society, and is more a dancer's curtsey than anything else. Curtseying to royalty was really the only time a deep curtsey was made, otherwise the head remained erect and tilted so as not to disturb the hairdressing. In stiff, high corsets it was impossible to bend far forward from the waist, and the bodice and sleeves fitted so tightly and exactly that the arms were restricted and could not be flung back like wings. The art of curtseying gracefully lay in the even sinking and rising without a prolonged pause to regain the balance while down.

Naturally, bows and curtseys were not only governed by period, but by the character of the part and degree of familiarity towards each other of those who used the greeting.

Curtsies in period costume were much easier than most amateurs imagine, and fall into two categories. A demure bending of both knee and head was correct from early Saxon times up to the seventeenth century, and can be used at any period when wearing either a very full skirt or even a crinoline.

Regency and Edwardian dresses needed a curtsey going down on one knee, as much or as little as the occasion demanded. If any deep curtsey was used, the supporting leg supported comfortably. If one knee was used, then they knelt firmly on it. If the deep stage curtsey is done, then sit on the underneath leg so that both thighs are supported. This makes it easy to gather the weight correctly for the ascent from the curtsey which is much harder to manage gracefully than the sinking.

Men's bows were intended to be courteous and, in any period when men's clothes were flamboyant, the bow should be so as well. An old man of any period naturally used the bow fashionable in his youth, and a countryman would also have used an old-fashioned reverence.

Informal bows were usually done with the feet together, care being taken not to drop the head so suddenly that the hat or wig dropped as well. Formal bows invariably had some type of preparatory step, forwards, sideways, or backwards, some amount of toe pointing, and a gesture of the hand towards the heart or the lady to whom the bow was made. Characterisation was shown in these formal manners almost as clearly as in the casual ones. Shaking hands nowadays is a formal gesture, but how very differently it is possible to perform it.

Stylised movement is dependent on the producer's wish, and can be used in any play: fantastic (*Prunella*), symbolic (*And so Ad Infinitum*), period (*The Beaux Stratagem, The Importance of being Earnest, Canterbury Tales*), or farce (*The Proposal*). It implies a precise pattern of movement both from individuals and from groups, in many cases coordinated with music, and always at a slightly different tempo from real life. Sometimes this tempo is slower, sometimes quicker, sometimes the actions will be very staccato, sometimes droopily wispy. Here is a brief example from John Clement's production of *The Beaux Stratagem*:

The three ladies were in the sitting-room, ready to go to church. Music was playing, and at a music cue they all took their parasols. As one woman they swung them up in front, opened them with a sharp click, twirled them on to their shoulders, and turned to face the window. A brief pause, then, one behind the other, they all started off simultaneously on the right foot and minced, in time with the music, out of the door, each parasol exactly at the same angle, in a stylised procession.

An example of where this type of movement is burlesqued is Gilbert and Sullivan's. Opera *Patience*.

Preliminary work on stylised movement should always be done with music to ensure exact timing. The hands are used from the wrists and elbows, rather than the shoulders, the legs use the knee angles persistently, the foot is either poised on the toe with knee bent, or on the heel, toe in the air, legs straight, the head angle is pronounced and the body angle more exaggerated than in everyday acting. This gives a rough idea, which is really all that can be done in a book. Stylised work must be recognised in order to be appreciated, but once the player has started on this habit of thought he will find it a fascinating study, with no holds barred. Ideas must be snatched from every source; ballet, pictures, old prints, any unusual position or variation of stance can be combined effectively. Even when playing modern farce, much of the movement is far from realism—for instance, pretending to be catching flies, when found out making a warning gesture to a friend. The double take, so familiar in films, when the comedian hears bad news with a happy smile, and then suddenly with his hands wipes the smile off his face, also qualifies as stylised gesture.

This type of gesture can be introduced in any particular way that the producer feels is consistent with the production. In burlesque stylised movement will probably be used throughout, but even in character comedy, speeches or short scenes, it could be used for a specific purpose.

Suppose that the young people in the play have offended someone, and are told they must all go and apologise. Instead of simply going out, all together, walking naturally, the leader would form the others into a small procession, giving each an appropriate classical mourning attitude, and then conducting them out, all wailing "Woe, Woe". This is a perfectly legitimate use of stylised movement, combining the underlining in a ridiculous way, of a trivial emotion, with a comedy effect of surprise. In this case the link with characterisation is that the scene is concerned with young people who tend to exaggerate.

Stylised movement is often used in verse plays; it sharpens the effect of elegance, heightens the effect of grotesquerie, and can gild the dull passage of words with visual glitter. In a curious way it lends an air of naturalness to movements in fantastic costumes, and shows them off to the best advantage, and a stylised position can be held for a length of time that would look awkward otherwise.

The difference between two people gossiping together in a natural position, or stylised, could be worked out in this way:

Realistic. Two elderly women in characteristic attitudes of a natural type would sit on two chairs which faced each other, but were probably not level with each other.
Stylised. The chairs would be placed centre stage, back to back, but slanted to make an angle, the women would both be knitting, holding their work high in front of them with elbows out, and each would turn her head sharply towards her neighbour as she spoke, and sharply back to her work as the other spoke.

Realistic. Two girls winding wool. One sits on a chair and holds the wool, the other sits on a footstool opposite and winds the wool into a ball. They change their positions slightly as they react to the emotions of the dialogue.
Stylised. One girl sits bolt upright, and winds the wool rhythmically, three quick winds and one sentence spoken, or line of verse, (phrase the rhythm as desired but keep it unvaried throughout). The other girl stands in a deep lunge as

in fencing, her upstage foot is forward and supported on footstool, knee bent; she is capable of swaying a long way to right or left as she looses the wool held in her outstretched hands. She can either sway in time to her words, and remain motionless while the other speaks, or vice versa.

The backs of the players can be far more often kept to the audience than in realistic movement, as a much sharper turn of head towards the audience can be used without looking out of place. In melodrama, with speeches of the "Little does he think" genre, this is obviously useful for the hero, while the heroine patters prettily down the buttercup field, and the villain slinks stealthily to his dastardly rendezvous.

Amateur men actors usually need much prodding before they will use these movements, but it is worth while goading them unmercifully as they are invariably excellent when they finally realise that the producer is adamant. In the right play a stylised fight can be infinitely funnier than a realistic one, whether duel, fists, or sticks are used. It is permissible to drop into slow motion to indicate the state of mind of one who gets stunned, or to quicken the movement ridiculously to convey time passing too rapidly towards an unwelcome event.

While movement may be mixed in this way and still be stylised, a period play performed with exaggerated modern poses, crinolined ladies smoking and crossing their legs, comes more under the heading of "Burlesque". Occasionally a position will be realistic if only used by one person, but become stylised if copied by two or more people at the same moment, with exaggerated tempo.

The fault to be guarded against is that of being too whimsical: the movement should sharpen the impact of the play and never in any circumstances blur it.

CHAPTER V

EXERCISE AND EXPERIMENT

THE *aim* of these exercises is to give the player in the shortest time, and with economy of effort, sufficient control over his body to enable him to use it as an instrument to its fullest extent. He can consult books on physical culture to develop muscles, suppleness and strength; the movements given now combine to make a short cut for actors. Individuals with special shortcomings, bow legs or tight Achilles tendons, will have to do special work. The average performer will find the following an interesting test of his own shortcomings and capabilities.

Each exercise combines several types of movement, to economise in time; it is hoped that students will work out their own variations on the lines suggested.

Any difficulty experienced while doing these is a sign that a particular part of the body needs special stretching. Probably most people will have sufficient recollection of school gym to correct their own failings, once they have discovered which they are.

It is helpful beyond words if at least two people can work together. Practising alone needs great strength of mind, and may easily be useless if the person has not a good eye to see exactly what is happening. An observer, not too carpingly critical, is needed, who will say whether the arm is really fully stretched. Some of these exercises are deliberately planned for two people, although easily done with an imaginary partner. The children's drill of sitting utterly motionless without even the eyes moving, for one, two, or three minutes, has defeated many an adult. Without someone else to watch one, it is fatally easy to cheat.

Limbering exercises, to stretch the muscles thoroughly, should always be done when the body is warm and relaxed, in fact directly on waking is a good time, or directly before going to sleep.

Deep breathing is the classic remedy for stage fright, but many victims are so tied up in knots that they can only breathe in shuddering gasps with their hearts thudding in their throats. Let them, in company with another sufferer, try Exercise 5; the concentration needed, and the sight of another person struggling with balance, is a sedative for nerves.

Head posture troubles many people, and the simplest exercise is as follows:

Hunch both shoulders up to the ears, draw the shoulder blades together, drop them firmly and jiggle them rather as if scratching the back against a post.

In doing all these exercises be precise in finding out exactly where they catch the muscles. Not just "in the back", localise it to the neck, shoulders, waist, or to thigh, knee or ankle. Then concentrate for a time with special exercises for that part, checking up regularly with the original exercise until it is easily repeated.

The following *problems* also arise.

There is no age limit for achievement: one gentleman of 74, with not much difficulty but steady persistence, corrected some very stiff leg movements, while another of 63 with a moderate amount of practise was able to enjoy more freedom of head movement than he had ever had in his life before.

One often sees sportsmen who have excelled in the field, hopelessly clumsy and unco-ordinated on the stage, and marvelled at the transformation. This is, however, mental, not really physical. Part of the perfect physical co-ordination achieved in sport comes from self-confidence, and this is often lacking when the sportsman tackles acting, as he feels he is out of his element. He must be shown as quickly and concisely as possible on what grounds the two elements, his own, and the stage, meet; and how they can be combined to his advantage. Self-confidence can be built up readily in this way, and the accumulated skill and dexterity developed by years of practice used to its best advantage. The time spent on various sports in summer should not be regarded by amateurs as time wasted away from acting, but used for the double purpose of their own enjoyment, and as a contribution to their art in acting.

Professionals can give their whole energy to their training, and then collapse, worn out, in the evening. The problem of the amateur is to use to the best advantage the time left over from his own job. Many excellent methods are, therefore, automatically ruled out as they would take more time and energy than is feasible. This is a point to which special attention has been given in the form of exercises that can be done at odd moments of waiting, and suggestions for concentrating on particular failings if there is not enough free time to correct everything. Any form of un-theatrical physical activity helps immensely when the Mr. George realises how to adapt it to his stage activity and does so consciously. The ball games— football, tennis, squash, and netball, all use intricate footwork, co-ordination of simultaneous body, foot, and head movement, and accurate judging of distance in a certain prescribed stage which can be used to great advantage in theatrical work. Hockey, cricket, and ping-pong require the use and control of the back and waist muscles, although the stooping posture is apt to become a bad habit. Boxing, with its skilled footwork, skating, with its perfect balance; climbing, which uses every muscle, swimming and diving, with their directed force of effort, will all add appreciably to the amateur's physical equipment for acting. Sir Frank Benson, in his company, laid great emphasis on the value of sport (other things being equal), and it is on record that what tipped the scale in the favour of one actress's engagement was that she had won a tennis tournament in the north of England. Any producer would have a right to expect better fencing in a Laertes who boxed than in one who did tapestry work.

Exercises for the hand and wrist are included which can be done at odd moments. A great deal of time can be used for exercises without putting aside a special hour, if waiting time is pressed into service. Waiting for a kettle to boil, for a bus to come, for a telephone kiosk to empty are all frustrating experiences which can be put to good account, and it is quite astonishing how the time mounts up in a week or two. Exercises should never be continued until one is tired and aching, they should be done just long enough to achieve further dexterity and a feeling of smugness.

Hand Exercises. Clench the hand as tightly as possible with the thumb outside, and spread the fingers, straightening them while stretching an imaginary octave. Clench the hand again tightly, with the thumb inside, then straighten the fingers, holding them closely together and pushing out the palm— try to make a hollow with the back of the hand to finish.

Place the finger tips on any surface (if sitting in a 'bus it can be done on the knees) and raise each finger separately as far as it will go and then tap it sharply back again as in typing. Let the arms hang down and the wrist go as far back as possible—rather like the comedy gesture of asking for a tip—then turn it as far as possible in the other direction. Bend the wrist at right angles to the arm so that the palm of the hand faces the floor, then bend it so that the back of the hand faces the floor.

The following exercises all look most peculiar if not insane, but just remember they are not meant for the on-looker but for the executant. It is quite easy to detach any particular movement from any exercise and do that one alone.

EXERCISE 1. *Stretching, Twisting, Relaxing*

Standing with the feet apart, stretch with the arms and fingers, turn the body to the right, stretch up, relax, and sweep the arms at full length round to the left, parallel with the ground, bending from the waist. Let this swing sweep the right foot off the floor, and carry the impetus on until the right foot is on the ground facing the opposite direction from the starting one. Repeat in the opposite direction.

EXERCISE 2. *Suppleness, Control, and Balance*

Kneel down with the arms stretched out to the side, sit back on the heels, place the hands on the floor behind the hips, release the right leg and stretch high in front, do the same with the left leg, pull up the feet to cross leg position, release the hands, and rise to a standing position.

EXERCISE 3. *Co-ordination, Accuracy, and Stretching*

Stand in a deep lunge on the left foot, stretch out both arms to the left, bring the arms and weight over to the right and stretch up, drawing a figure of eight in front, the starting position making the bar in the centre of the eight.

EXERCISE 4. *Lightness and Elasticity*

With both feet together, bounce on the balls of the feet, increase the bounce in height, then change on to alternate feet, finally with the knees bending gradually more and more until sitting on the haunches.

EXERCISE 5. *Flexibility of Neck and Spine*

Stand with the back to a table, drop the head back as far as possible, chew an imaginary bar of gum, while drawing the knee up to the waist in front with both hands clasping it, straighten the leg out in front, and hold for two counts before replacing it on the floor.

EXERCISE 6. (*To be done in Couples.*)

Stand facing each other, palm to palm at arm's length from each other, A lunges forward while B lunges back, both stretching arms and spine as much as possible and using rotary head movements. Without recovering to starting position B immediately lunges forward while A lunges back. Practise this first in a straight line, and then travelling round in a circle.

EXERCISE 7. (*To be worked out by Students*)

In order that stretching should never be done vaguely, three variations are given for students to work out in their own way, so at to concentrate the work on their own personal problems. Choose a letter, a number, or geometrical shape. Stand with feet apart and arms stretched facing an imaginary wall, draw on it any letter of the alphabet, assuming it to be at head height. Use the full stretch of both arms, bend both knees to a kneeling position to stand the letter on the floor, twist from the waist if it has a bar across as in A. The value of imagining a letter lies in the fact that the exercise will have clarity and precision and exploit the muscles stretched to the fullest capacity. Repeat the movement, drawing a star. Then repeat it drawing a number.

Finally, remember the qualities that need to be developed in the body, and adopt any means that will lead to achieving them or that solves any unusual individual difficulty.

The body in its entirety (head, arms and legs) should be flexible, controlled, sensitive and expressive, a docile instrument capable of doing effortlessly anything the part demands. Amateurs need not feel that they are thwarted by not being able to give their full time to the stage, if they remember time has to be spent studying characters in real life before they can be translated into theatrical terms. If they practise walking in a poised and easy way in their every-day lives, they will not need to worry about lack of time to practise walking on the stage; they will simply proceed as usual.

PART TWO

THE CROWD

CHAPTER VI

THE EXTERNAL APPROACH

THIS Part deals entirely with the external approach to stylised plays, pageants, etc. It is emphatically not a method to be advised for children. Its uses are:

1. For adults and particularly for *Youth Clubs*, where self-consciousness has to be overcome.

2. For pageants where acting is on a broad scale and large numbers of actors are concerned.

3. For religious plays where the sincere and genuine emotion of those taking part can be utterly ruined by clumsy positions, and where the actor can be freed from worry only if the framework is exact.

Again it is stressed that this book aims at giving a framework on which to build without having to start with the foundations each time. The method is explained in detail for uses with the first group mentioned above.

This form of stylised movement consists of the *imposing of a pattern* entirely *by the producer*. He uses his players pictorially, building up his groups with arrangements of bodies, angles of heads, arms or legs, and without imposing any emotional demands on his actors. He will arrange his actors in attitudes of fear, create a group that denotes horror, or a motionless row of people who convey despair; but it is done physically not mentally. The fascinating part of this method is the way it can overcome the most stubborn forms of shyness and self-consciousness.

The pattern made by the body creates its own mental image in the most impressive way. Being placed by the producer in a stylised position, at a particular angle, with even the method of progression dictated (eight slow walks, pause, all round the stage), relieves the self-conscious one of a large load of personal responsibility. Released from the fear of showing off or doing something silly (in fact giving herself away), entirely covered by the producer's instructions, she will unconsciously find herself feeling the emotions her body is expressing.

The Expressionistic Method would start this way:

"Express fear" says the producer. The unhappy victim sees three choices. She can giggle weakly, she can attempt to do what is wanted and succeed only in expressing acute embarrassment, or she can be sick on the spot and never act again. Her own personal choice, which would be to sink through the floor, is rarely practical.

Now for the External Method:

"Six of you stand here", says the producer, "shoulder to shoulder, alternately facing outward and inward, in a diamond formation. Now turn in the left toe until it touches the other instep, bending the knees slightly. Raise the right shoulder and bring the right hand across the body to hold the left elbow, turn your head over the right shoulder while still looking in front of you."

By now, although it is dictated slowly and each order is followed before the next is issued, Miss Georgina has not had much time to think of herself. Everyone else is getting into the same position, she does not yet know what character she is, what emotion, if any, she will have to display, but (and this is the important point) she has not yet been asked to do anything she feels she cannot do, and her self-confidence, therefore, is being built up.

"Now," says the producer, "when the music starts I

will count two and clap my hands. It does not matter if you do not all start together, but start as soon as you can. I want you to shuffle round the stage keeping in your diamond shape until you come back to where you started. Then I want you to shuffle inwards until you are a tight little wad all pressed closely together. The ones facing outwards will shuffle backwards at this point, and those facing inwards will shuffle forwards, and the music will go on until you are all close together."

The group do this, sometimes seriously, sometimes with relieved giggles at finding they really can do it. They know where they are going, they know they are doing it properly, they do not yet know why, nor what the effect is supposed to be. They have now, however, mastered the mechanics sufficiently to be able, and to want, to go on to something further.

"This time", says the producer, "you are going to do it without any help from me in starting you. So I will help you in another way. You are meant to be a group of frightened and hopeless people. You are driven out of your homes, you do not know where to go, you only have each other and huddle together for comfort, in a sort of dreary dream. You know exactly what to do, you would probably be wearing rags, and we might play it with a blue light, and wind howling."

He has not, please notice, asked them to express anything at all, even now. He has given them a clear mental picture of what they ought to look like, and clear, practical instructions of how to look like it.

By now, relaxed and interested and not being under the necessity to do any more (such is the infallible contrariness of human nature), any group, almost without exception, buckles to and projects all the misery and hopelessness that any producer can wish.

In a cramped position, with twisted head and huddled body, tied down by shuffling steps and restricted to a close formation, it would be indeed an actress worth hailing who could express joy in these circumstances.

The foregoing is an example of how the method works; and that it does work has been proved most satisfactorily, both with tough groups and with genteel groups.

It is not, of course, the only method with self-conscious groups, but it is quick and sound in its results. It lays a firm foundation of practical knowledge and its practical application, which are the deadly enemies of self distrust. So much concentration is clearly needed to follow the exact instructions, that there is little or no time to worry about feelings. The instructions mastered, confidence gathers and with it the desire to master something more. Not something of a different element, something more of the same type. It is most important, if the thing is approached from this angle, to be consistent.

The producer should tell the groups about the emotions at the moment he deems fit. Sometimes this is after they have repeated the movement twice, sometimes much more repetition is necessary. Sometimes it can be done quite near the beginning of a class or rehearsal, occasionally it has to be left to the end.

The teacher or producer is the person to gauge whether the group is still clinging to the safety of obeying orders, or whether it is slightly impatiently waiting to be told why it is doing the exercise.

It is better to keep the students working in groups, practically anonymously until they are ready to emerge as individuals. When this time comes the producer continues in exactly the same way, with every attitude clearly mapped out, specific instructions for each move, and exact time of start and finish. No emotion is attempted until the character is ready to express it, and is in the right position to do so.

Here follow two *practical examples* of this method used in co-ordination with words and music:

A. Explain the scene from *Abraham Lincoln* where the negro, alone in Lincoln's office, listens to the soldiers passing the window, marching to free his fellow slaves, and then bursts into tears.

The negro stands by the window, arms spread, hands resting on the sill, looking out until he watches the soldiers go round the corner. Then he transfers the weight of his body to the right foot, slides his right hand up the window frame so that his head can rest on it and lets the left arm drop by his side. At no time is his face seen by the audience.

The soldiers stand on one side, out of sight. Theoretically they are marching down the street towards the window, singing "John Brown's Body" and turning the corner fading away in the distance. Appoint a leader and let all start marching and singing a verse of the song. The volume increases slowly until on the second "Glory, Glory, Halleluia" the peak is reached when presumably they are just outside the window, from then song and marching come more and more faintly until they die away.

Points to notice:

1. Marching must not quicken as song grows louder.
2. Marching steps must keep time with song.
3. Climax of sound must come from everyone.
4. Dying away must not be too sudden.

At first this will all be very raggedly done, but it is so obvious when all is not well that the students are eager to correct themselves and try again. Do this in two groups, if possible, letting each learn from the other's mistakes.

Those least in need of this method and most advanced in their ideas of acting will always volunteer to be the negro, and should be encouraged to take individual parts in the other exercises.

B. WITCH HUNT. To be done with background music; spontaneous dialogue can be introduced either before the crowd starts to move or during the progression towards the Witch.

PATTERN. The Witch sits down-stage left, her back to entrance which is up-stage right, crouched over fire. The crowd is arranged in three diagonal lines one behind the other, the tallest members in the back line, the largest number in the middle line.

STEPS. Back line footwork: side L., close R., side L., starting with left foot, travelling rapidly towards the Witch and back again towards the group. They cover the distance about three times as often as the middle group, their arms outspread, beckoning to the others. The middle group stand shoulder to shoulder in a wedge-shaped block, facing front, heads turned towards left shoulder, right hand holding left elbow. Their step is: side, close, side, close, done in very small shuffles. The group must stay in close formation and move in a cramped and contorted way to express an ugly emotion.

The third group, which should not consist of more than two people, do the same step as the first group, but using very little space, they start after the other two groups are a third of the way across the stage, their arms hang loosely, their heads are dropped, but their eyes watch the Witch. This is the group which wants to join in but holds back. The first two groups travel until they completely surround the Witch and hide her, and then hold their positions. As the Witch screams, they all sink to their knees and stretch arms up and forward, elbows bent and fingers crooked as if for tearing. The third group stands slightly to one side and turns away, flinging up their elbows to cover their eyes.

Points to notice:

The back line must move very quickly, using huge steps so that it flickers like a flame between the Witch and the others. The second line must fix their eyes on the Witch, raise their left shoulder and keep steadily moving without losing formation. All must finish with faces hidden. Climaxes of horror are always a bugbear to selfconscious groups who invariably give way to laughter out of sheer embarrassment; therefore exercises of this sort should be planned so as to put as little strain as possible on the actors facial control.

Work of this sort must be planned beforehand by a producer thoroughly conversant with the method, it cannot be attacked in the same way as Improvised or Spontaneous Drama.

There are many sources from which to get material for exercises, and it is often successful to ask the class, or group, to suggest something for next time. In most cases they suggest something that they have heard on the wireless which needs a good deal of imagination to transpose into visual drama. It is wise to encourage any suggestions from the group, either as to material, steps, pace, music, or grouping, as it is much easier to instruct Youth Groups especially by the question and answer method. They will listen cheerfully and intelligently to a comparatively long and involved answer to a direct question, but not be able to concentrate for the same length of time on something the producer has decided to teach them. Also, if anyone shows an inclination towards producing a short scene in this manner, let him be given a definite scene, cast, and time limit, but do not let anyone try to arrange anything on the spur of the moment. To work out moves properly in this way there must be time to study the possible contrasts needed, and select the rhythms and steps; it defeats its own end if hasty and slovenly work is permitted.

When the group has gained sufficient confidence to advance into individual work, occasionally some movement studies may be given, the students working in pairs. *The Insect Play* could be briefly explained and each pair work out a type of progression suitable for whatever insect it wishes to choose. This gives enormous scope, some couples move across the stage squatting on the heels, some trip with outstretched wings, and some progress in a series of leaps. The pair may make either similar movements, exactly reversed movements, or complementary ones. One pair demonstrated a Beetle Husband and Wife in such an exercise, by the husband scuttling forward and sawing the air with both hands as he obviously laid down the law in high chirruping accents. His beetle wife followed slightly behind him, taking a zig-zag course, and nodding her head in meek agreement as she drew level with him at each point of her zig-zag.

Students are unexpectedly fertile in ideas if they are not allowed to have any initiative until the end of the session, but it is hopeless to expect them to do anything at the beginning of the session or after a pause, in cold blood. If possible let the suggestions be concentrated on one particular aspect each time. First try changes in the tempo of the various steps used, and let the students experiment until they see why certain steps are effective when done quickly and not when done slowly. Next time experiment with the type of step used, the time after that with lines of direction and pattern. This brings to the fore the question as to why some patterns are dramatic when done by twenty people, and dull when done by only one. It can be shown how an exhilarating effect can be obtained with flowing curves and raised lines, and a depressing one by crooked lines and cramped crowds.

The reason for this method must never be lost to sight, therefore the time for students' suggestions must not be allowed to encroach on the training time. It must be kept as an exciting finish to the session or even as an incentive to the work, never taken for granted. Much time can be delightfully wasted while students clutch their heads for the brilliant idea they have "almost got"! This is why emphasis has been laid on the fact that any complete scene must be planned outside class time.

The *dialogue* used can either be a scene from a play, a prose passage from the Bible, *Pilgrim's Progress*, *Treasure Island*, or any other suitable book, poetry or blank verse from any suitable source or naturalistic conversation supplied by the cast, but *not improvised during the movement*. When the last-mentioned alternative is chosen, the scene must be explained and plot lines and character lines allocated, with the characters repeating the exact words. These may be provided either by themselves or the producer, but they must be set and not made up as they go along. It needs a rather advanced group to do this successfully and keep the timing and movement clear-cut and accurate. Poetry is a risky thing and should have a strong rhythm or a repeated refrain. The wise producer will read it first to his flock, and if he sees any signs of shrinking on their part, remark casually, "We might do that another time." He can then bring up the subject some sessions later and see if the response is the same, and if it is, then poetry can be scratched off the list. There are some items in this method that the producer must set his teeth and carry through, willy-nilly, but poetry should not be one of them. At the same time it is such a useful and inspiring medium that it must be given at least two fair chances before being abandoned.

The Psalms are nearly always popular with Youth Groups, and produce some most unexpected suggestions and results when selected as homework.

A time will come when it is advisable for the class to split into two groups, and compete with each other. This is a very critical moment as they are near the time when they will no longer need the help of the external method.

Watching the second group do the exercises outlined in this chapter, it will be borne in on Group No. 1 what the vital factor is which will make them the better group. They will understand that in such a set piece there is nothing to stop either group being technically perfect, the means and the method are theirs. What will make the better performance is, obviously, how much more vividly one group projects the feeling and emotion than the other. They will then understand how important the outward shell is, but also how limited if there is nothing in it.

Once they have not only realised this but applied it, they can pass out of this group and take their place, confidently, among their fellow actors.

CHAPTER VII

STYLISED CROWD SCENES

STYLISED crowd scenes are dependant on careful *design*, using floor pattern, a variety of steps and tempo, and simple but accurate positioning of the top half of the body and hands. Music and sound effects are attractive trimmings, but basically it should be possible to stop one's ears and watch a pleasing and exciting picture. It should also be possible at any given moment to have immobility and still see a pleasing design.

The first time a producer plans a stylised crowd it is as well to start with one long-suffering individual. Let the producer push this person into different positions and attitudes, making a note of all the effective and useful ones. He should work downward from the head, through shoulders, arms, knees, and feet, until he is quite sure what particular positions will make the pattern. He can then work out the different positions and placings on the stage.

A crowd wedged together tightly need only move their heads to express fright, and one arm which is laid along the shoulder of the nearest neighbour can be multiplied by twenty to make a design.

Another crowd, scattered over the stage, wearing long cloaks, may use their cloaks in unison, swinging their arms like windmills and travelling over the stage in a wedge-shaped formation. If fantastic costume is to be worn, position and gesture should be planned accordingly and the floor pattern fitted in afterwards. If the crowd is drably dressed, the floor pattern comes first and dictates the steps and places. If the crowd scene finishes on a note of appeal, with a beggar flinging up his arms, he must be given a leaping step in the plan so that he can leap on to the rostrum at the vital moment.

Few things need more care than planning a stylised crowd scene, and in this chapter is given a practical method for varying the treatment according to the size of the crowd, stage, and type of play. It may look intimidating in cold print, but immediately it is worked out with humans the pattern will fall into place and difficulties will be overcome.

Floor patterns can be visualised quite simply by imagining that the performers have wet bare feet and are leaving footprints. The simplest way of drawing them is by a line with arrows at intervals showing the direction the steps are taking. Coloured pencils to indicate the different steps used, or the tempo, can help; red can be used, for instance, for quick running steps, blue for slow marches. Some prefer to do the floor pattern in black, with arrows in colour to show the speed, and a coloured line by the black one to show the steps used. Sometimes one wants to change the step or the tempo but not the direction, and this method makes an alteration easy. It is quite clear to see when one makes a plot of this sort, whether the pattern is dull or interesting, repetitive or contrasting.

The design should not be done only in circles; but diagonal lines, zig-zags, semi-circles, triangles, squares, straight lines crossing, stars and rosettes are all useful and decorative. Study the following which are group formations:

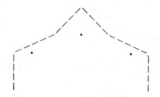

A. The unbroken angles can be achieved by the actors putting hands on each other's shoulders, the dot effect by them standing at attention or kneeling.

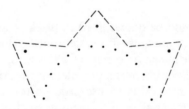

B. The semi-circle of dots are actors sitting cross-legged, the three large dots are actors standing, and the back angles are formed with actors carrying banners.

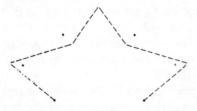

C. The angles here are formed by actors kneeling on one or both knees and the dots are actors standing upright with swords raised in salute.

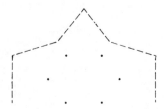

D. Formation for a religious play; outside actors standing
   solidly shoulder to shoulder, facing towards centre group,
   with hands crossed on breast. Centre group facing outwards with hands in praying position at waist. Heads of
   outside group bent, of inside group raised to heaven. All
   standing with feet closely together.

These could be drawn in plain black as they are static
groups, but sometimes it is easier to use a different colour
for each character or group of characters, e.g, blue for
angels, pink for cherubs and violet for the Angel Gabriel.

Another method is to use little postcard men with a
bit of the material of the costume stuck on them, but
eventually the group must be drawn for rehearsals and
the prompt copy, with consideration for the dimensions
of the stage.

The difference between a large stage and a small stage
must be taken into account in planning steps. If A has
eight quick steps to get to the throne, and B eight slow
ones it must be quite certain A can do this in eight and
only eight. For a simple move on a large stage this is not
important, but for concerted movement on a small stage
it is absolutely vital.

An interweaving pattern demands that each individual
shall be in exactly the same place, at the same moment,
each time he rehearses. A satisfactory pattern can be made
working from one entrance, and duplicating from the
other entrance, each group using half the stage. If one is

tired or rushed it is feasible to take a plan one has used before and reverse it. If the design was straight lines and triangles in quick tempo, one would have curves and circles in slow tempo. Crowd scenes planned this way obviate the usual milling to and fro, with uneasy smiles on meeting the same people perpetually, that inexperienced producers find difficult to avoid.

Take a stage with two down-stage entrances and two up-stage, and a crowd of villagers "revelling":

A and B enter together up-stage right, make complete circle.

C and D enter together down-stage right, make complete circle, all using slow steps and pauses.

E enters down-stage left, crosses to up-stage entrance right, returns in diagonal line.

F enters up-stage right, crosses to down-stage entrance left, returns in diagonal line.

G enters up-stage left, makes zig-zag line across stage to down-stage and back.

H enters down-stage left, makes zig-zag line across stage to up-stage back centre.

I enters up-stage right, and weaving in and out, works his way back to his original entrance.

If E and F use a running step, G uses skips, H uses four skips and four runs, and I takes four steps forwards and turns, then does four steps backwards still travelling in the same direction, the pattern will be varied in line and tempo. The letter A can stand for one person or two, or a group.

The crowd can be prepared for this type of production by giving them walking exercises to music. of *varied rhythms*.

1. Two quick paces forward, pause two counts.
   Four slow paces forward, eight counts.
   To be done in 4/4 time, taking six bars.
2. Three quick paces forward, three counts pause and two slow paces. To be done in 3/4 time, taking four bars.

3. Three paces forward taken slowly, close feet on 4th. To be done in 3/4 time, taking four bars.

Exercise 2 can be done by two or four people travelling down-stage from centre entrance.

Exercise 3 to be done simultaneously by four people travelling round the stage clockwise, and four anti-clockwise, all starting from same entrance. Practise timing so that sometimes the group finishes up-stage and sometimes down.

In the beginning start all moving simultaneously, as they get more advanced teach them to take music cues and "stagger" the entrances. Occasionally plot the moves in slow time and bring in quick movers with just enough time to get into positions. A necessarily slow and unwieldy procession can have dramatic interest added to it in this way.

For small stages take the following exercise:

1. This one gives the effect of a long and stately procession but takes up less room. The actor moves a pace forward on his down-stage foot and brings his feet together, then a small pace to the side on his up-stage foot, and brings his feet together. The progression is: left foot forward, close right to left, *right* foot sideways, close left to right; he is then making a turreted floor pattern. If he keeps moving alternate feet, it would develop into a crab-like movement, so please study this carefully.

2. For a romantic Ruritanian procession in waltz time, couples travelling forward start facing forward, two steps forward (taking two bars), one small step backward (taking one bar), one small step forward (taking one bar). When the procession is composed of couples, men and women, or all women, *not* all men, variations can be used. The steps and timing exactly the same as before but the direction altered. Or, on the third and fourth step, instead of being side by side, the couple take abackward step away from each other, and then a forward step towards each other.

This type of thing can reduce the most pompous to baffled bewilderment, and the most rowdy Youth Club into shoving one another round the way wanted, not the way they want, but they quickly learn and it gives the producer the priceless asset of public opinion if they do get it wrong. Any member of a group, completely incapable of keeping in time himself, can yet unerringly, and vocally, notice if anyone else is a beat behind. There is an absolute standard of right and wrong, in time or out, far away from the feeling "the producer is being very fussy tonight". From the producer's view point it is infinitely easier to direct and watch than to do it oneself.

The patterns so far have all been made by plain walking steps, putting one foot in front of the other, which achievement one has the right to expect from an average performer. There are many other elementary movements which can be considered and used successfully to create dramatic effect, and which, when done unsuccessfully, will create a comedy effect.

Various simple steps are:

1. A simple skip (step on one foot and hop on same foot).

2. Running steps taken very lightly on the ball of the foot.

3. Hop on one foot, interpolated at regular intervals.

4. Three runs and one hop.

5. Eight runs and two hops.

6. For an agitated effect: run, and hop on counts three, seven, nine and eleven.

These can be practised in every direction including going backwards, which could be sub-titled "Chaos in Curves". It is wise to practise the steps separately very thoroughly indeed, before alternating them, as they are confusing to beginners in this work.

7. Gallop or slip step: such as is used in reels, travelling

sideways, the foot is taken to the side and with a slight bounce the other foot is brought up to it. Great speed can be attained with this step, without the same strain on the floorboards of the stage that quick skips would be. Psychologically, this is a good step with which either to wind up a class, or prepare for a new, difficult exercise, as it is most exhilarating for the performers. Dramatically it helps in scenes of orgies where the predominant note is not intended to be gentility. Done with bent knees the most restrained of players gives an impression of licentious abandonment. Some producers may have experienced difficulty in getting just this effect from worthy but inhibited players.

There are many other simple varieties of steps, but it is better to concentrate on a few steps, used with contrasting pace and pattern.

In plotting the pattern the physical peculiarities of your cast are also to be considered. With the same basic step four stout people can make a compact, reassuring block; four spindly, tall people can look uneasy and wavering; four massive, tall people can look downright bloodthirsty. Contrasting sizes can be used either pictorially or comically to build up your group, or to relieve tension. There is no question of certain steps suiting certain sizes; it entirely depends on the general effect wanted.

The use of different stage levels virtually depends on the stage carpenter, if the rostrum is diffident with only itself to support, it is obviously not going to take kindly to six deadly vices carousing on it. If a rostrum is only large enough to hold one character the movement could be restricted to the arms, body, and head, or possibly slow turns on the same spot. Stairs on the other hand, are usually well and solidly constructed and can be used effectively for pauses.

Psychologically, the confidence the players will get from moving easily and lightly up and down stairs that they themselves are convinced are going to collapse, will be invaluable to them at the moment the stairs actually do collapse. They will continue to move easily and lightly out of the debris, while every other producer in the audience is gnashing his teeth to know how that was done. Those plays which demand that the players enter through the aisles of the audience gain by this type of movement. Instead of a sheepish shuffle, bumping their elbows against the audience, they will carry the entrance through with an impetus that links it, in the right way, with what is happening on the stage.

Arena theatre gives a great opportunity for choreographic planning, mainly because the type of play suitable for arena work practically always has a large cast. The many entrances need the visual appeal of crowd work in the round grouping of either a highly stylised or violently naturalistic form. Individual characters will gain also from the balance and control these steps will build up. They make the rehearsals of crowd scenes far more interesting for the performers, there is not the same temptation to an actor to skip a rehearsal (because he is only one and will not be noticed) when he is kept hard at work learning the steps and formation. The producer will use his own judgement as to when he explains the meaning of the character and the scene.

CHAPTER VIII

EVERYDAY CROWDS

WHEN a producer has crowd scenes consisting of small-part characters, his task is a comparatively easy one, as he can count on the acting and merely has the grouping to arrange. *Realistic crowd scenes,* however, include those with "extras"—a large or small number of people who have no part in the play other than to be a crowd. Extras should know what the play is about and tackle their parts in exactly the same way as Mr. George. Their individual acting, though, must be more subordinated to the general mood of the scene. No extra should hold the attention of the audience for too long, or distract attention from the parts which have significance in the play. The audience should not be compelled to waste time watching someone who does not further the play in any way. While thus occupied, something else of importance may not be noticed. Also, if an audience gets interested in a character and then finds that person has no further part in the play it feels thwarted.

In real life, the fact that the crowd consisted of courtiers and noblemen rather than an uneducated rabble would make a certain difference from the point of view of movement. On the stage the difference is lessened, and for theatrical purposes the mass effect is the same. There is merely the elimination of any plebeian gestures that individuals may be using, such as wiping a mouth on a sleeve. The general bearing will be more dignified and upright for a crowd of nobles, and the general effect of more weighty authority, however excited they are about their rights. There is, for instance, a very different head tilt used by the man who says defiantly, "I got my rights, aint I?" and the man who says, "Of course I have my rights!"

Masking, or blocking another actor from the audience's sight, is something about which the producer will give orders, but it is a firm responsibility for each individual actor. There may be crowd scenes in which everyone has to be closely huddled together to make a mass of bodies. In this case Mr. George must huddle closely, not allowing daylight to be seen between him and his neighbours. In other scenes, every member of the crowd has a separate function, and the producer will dress the stage, showing each of his cast to the best advantage. It is then Mr. George's job to see that he is in the completely correct spot on the stage, and if he is blocked by anyone, to shift slightly until he can be seen by the audience. It is the responsibility of the up-stage actor not to let himself be masked—he cannot expect the down-stage actor to look round to see if anyone is lurking behind him.

Crowd scenes usually mean that the function of the crowd is to build up some form of *emotional climax*—therefore too much characteristic gesture will dull the general effect. Occasionally a producer will keep one character detached from the emotion, continuing his usual pursuits on one side of the stage as a contrast, but that is the producer's choice, not the actor's. In such scenes, as always, the individual responsibility still rests with the actors; the responsibility for the dramatic effect of the scene, with the producer. In Sean O'Casey's play *Red Roses for Me* , a scene has to be played on the bridge of a river— the bridge running across the back of the stage from side to side, and a row of characters lounging against it. In such a scene one is often presented with a line of hunched backs and drooping trouser seats, which are boring and repetitive. To tackle a crowd of this sort, survey first the possibility of using the scenery. Suppose there are eight men to be placed along the bridge. Nos. 1 and 2 could sit on the top of the parapet, leaning their backs to support each other; No. 3 could sit on the ground, leaning his back against the parapet at the other end of the bridge. No. 4 leans with his back against the bridge, his arms stretched full length along it, one hand just above No. 3 sitting on the ground; No. 5 is turned sideways, his elbow on the parapet but by No. 4's outstretched hand, and No. 6 is standing closely behind smoking. Thus, then, is the group of six at one end of the bridge—all linked together. At the other end No. 7 is standing with his back to the audience, looking at the river; No. 8 is standing sideways, one foot resting on a small ledge, his hand resting on the shoulder of the man next to him, No. 7. With the exception of the man on the ground (and he can easily get up) they can all look either into the river, or at anything that may be going on elsewhere. The monotonous effect previously mentioned sometimes arises from the following fact. If the scene is one in which "extras" are all meant to be miserable, out of work and hopeless, each person will use the same physical attitude to express the mood; and the producer will not have time to cope with each separately. Of course, he should make time, but this is where one comes up against the fact of the real versus the ideal. While this rearranging lies really in the producer's province, Mr. George would be well advised to glance around him to see if his own position is being duplicated by anyone else, and if so, to change it. He must realise the acute difference between this and a stylised crowd scene, where he may have to duplicate everything about his position, to that of his neighbours, even to the raising of one eyebrow. It is much quicker and easier for a producer to say "Don't do that", than for him to show how it should be done. Mr. George must still try to work out his own attitudes. Many of the same principles apply to arranging a realistic crowd scene as to a stylised crowd scene, but the question of *stage levels* is far more acute. If the stage is built up on several levels it is a comparatively simple affair, but if the stage is flat, whether large or small, it is one of the most difficult problems a producer can have. It is so much easier to get variety when there is liberty to use stylised positions, and arbitrarily put a row of actors cross-legged to clear the sight lines.

In order to get away from all the heads being at the same level, one must use outside help, as well as floor plans. Very high heels on some, flat heels on others, crutches, sticks (which can be clutched with both hands while the owner bends right forward over it), roller skates, stilts, bathchairs, wheelchairs, etc., can all be pressed into service according to the size of the stage and the type of crowd. If there is a newspaper boy, let him have a box on which two people can stand at the height of the excitement. If it topples and they fall off together, this can be timed for the best moment when it will add to the general excitement. A man can kneel down to tie his shoelace and stay on the edge of the crowd in that position, if the focus of the scene is on hearing something rather than seeing it. Small people can climb pick-a-back on their friends' backs. Women can stand with their backs to the centre of attraction, holding their handbag mirrors in the air to act as periscopes. It is not always effective to see the faces of the crowd—a forest of raised hands indicates just as clearly that there is a crowd.

Even with realistic crowds, the movement marked as "they all stream across the stage towards the strike breakers" does not mean that each person should run in a straight line towards the objective, all starting together as a race does. They should each be given a separate line, some straight, some more curved than others, and, like rays, converge on to the objective. Pace must be varied, but as it must appear headlong, the reason for the slowness of some must be obvious to the audience. Blind, lame, or old people cannot move so quickly, and are candidates for the slowest steps and the shortest line of advance. Some runner can make a detour to give the illusion of racing, and a few can run back again rapidly to call in others. Playing with crowds is a fascinating game, but it must not become too absorbing. In several recent productions, the crowd scenes have been so intricately planned that the eye of the audience was continually led away from the focal point. This should not happen, above all when the crowd is meant to be realistic. It is a pattern of the wrong sort when the audience is distracted by watching one actor worm his way purposefully across stage during an orator's speech until the big moment when he has to catch the flung-away cloak. Such business is better given to someone standing closely by the orator. A crowd at the beginning of a fair scene, which perhaps has to hold the stage during some dull and unimportant opening dialogue, may well have an intricate pattern, vivid characterisation, and a certain amount of by-play. A crowd which exists merely to project a mob emotion must subordinate all these things to this one end, and never cause an audience to wonder which part of the stage it ought to be watching. Many scenes are played with the crowd in a little clot round the focal character. Much ingenuity is sometimes used to arrange them so as not to become just a display of backs, when the producer would be better employed in considering the fundamental point of the episode. If the value of the crowd is in its ability to focus attention on the main character, and to *listen* to what he is saying, it is not necessary to press closely round him. The scene could just as well be arranged with the stage nicely dressed all over. The main point is that everyone should *look* as if they were listening intently, and this can be done by arranging for all heads to be turned towards the speaker, and for the actors furthest away from him to lean forward, which they can easily do, even if they are sitting down. Cliché grouping should be avoided as a rule, and only relied upon if, after earnest self-questioning, one decides that it is the only way. If it is only the best way, still, it is often more dramatically effective to choose some other alternative. One can lose the interest of the audience by showing them something so familiar that it has ceased to move them.

A very brief word about "*falls*" in crowds, which should always be strongly characterised—some people allow themselves to faint, others fight against faintness, for instance. A fall forward might be because of tripping over an obstruction, or because of being coshed from behind. The mechanics of any actor's fall must obviously be to ensure that he is not hurt, and can continue to act, if he has to, later on in the play. Few people, after they are two or three years old, are able to relax completely and fall so that they are not hurt. A fall must be relaxed, but controlled so that the floor hits those parts of the body protected by fleshy padding. These are: the back of the shoulders, the back of the hip, and the back of the calf. Forward falls usually need some cheating; they start forward, twist to hit the parts mentioned, and can finish with a roll into forward, backward, or sideways positions. Never let the head bounce with a sharp crack on the floor; or fall on to a straight arm or wrist, unless it is not necessary to play again for some weeks.

If a crowd has to fall in a heap, one on top of the other, care must be taken as to how this is to be done. Build it up from one person's fall, and plan which bit of each person falls on which bit of anyone else. Black eyes are not easily avoided if such falls are left to chance. Again, the effect may be simultnaeous, but the falls should be timed to have a split second between each. Start by making the crowd stand in a straight line, and fall in a straight line. It can then be seen which of them know how to fall, and which of them can control the exact direction in which they fall.

Warn them that they will have to fall three times in a line before they are trusted to fall in a heap. This saves recriminations later on, and enables it to be seen whether the fall is really controlled, or whether the first one was a fluke. If two are really hopelessly bad, let them drop on their knees, and slither forwards to lie on their faces.

CHAPTER IX

RELIGIOUS DRAMA

THE main problems of movement in Religious Drama are provided by the parish players, production in churches, and the ultra-modern play.

One of the greatest problems the producer has to face is a group consisting of a cross-section of Church members. The *Parish Players* are nobly prepared to do their duty, sincere and willing to learn. They are not, however, all attracted by the idea of acting, as is the case of the average amateur society. Therefore they will need a great deal more teaching, and precise explanation of what the producer wants. It is best to divide the group at the casting rehearsal into those who want to act and those who are there as loyal parishioners. These people will usually find dramatic speech and singing much easier than any form of dramatic movement. They must be helped in every way possible. Special coaching should be given, and movements and positions arranged that are well within their scope. They will find it easy to move convincingly as shepherds, merchants, native sellers or water carriers. They should not be given a part which needs difficult gesture if it is to be put across correctly. They can be cast as angels who process, or stand still, but not as angels who have to use sweeping arm gestures with conviction and finality.

With such people self-consciousness is not the basic cause of their difficulty, therefore stylised movement is not the best solution. They are performing an act of worship, in a manner imposed on them by a sense of duty, and are therefore ready to subdue their own feelings for the good of the cause. They need to be freed mentally from the fear of blundering physically. Only then will they be able to make a full contribution to the spiritual offering.

In all religious drama the spiritual effort given out by the players is so intense that many of their physical problems are solved in a way that is little short of miraculous. The producer very seldom has to bother about getting the right mood for this or that scene. On the contrary, the emotional feeling sometimes pours out so strongly that rather than having to work to extract it from the group, he will be more likely to need to check it to prevent it from becoming sentimental. This sentimentality more usually expresses itself in the voice than in the movement; but in either case it must be firmly suppressed.

Some simple relaxing exercises should always start the rehearsal, so that the players can move freely and comfortably by the time they are called upon to take up their parts. It is sometimes a little difficult to make such a group see that sincerity is not enough, that in a dramatic production the sense of drama must be preserved. The producer must also look at it from their point of view, and realise that anything too far from their usual routine will distract their minds from worship. He must hold the balance even more carefully than usual between his play production and his players.

The second problem he has is the question of *Production in Churches*. It should be obvious that not all religious plays are suitable to be performed in churches, but many seem unable to grasp this fact. Sometimes the reason the play is unsuitable is the theme, sometimes the difficulty is the technical one of stage craft. It is seldom satisfactory to transfer a stage production to a church, or vice versa. The production should be planned from the beginning either as a church production or not, irrespective of whether any particular church is chosen for the presentation.

Religious plays combine more possibilities of different

types of groups than perhaps any other class of play. There are not only shepherds, nobles and saints, but also angels of all sizes, with their contrasting wings. There are the angles of crooks, banners, haloes and spears to work into designs of richness or simplicity. The producer has it in his power to choose almost any pattern he feels will interpret the play, with the certainty that he has the material with which to display it. Religious paintings of the early centuries show an immense variety of position and groupings. The composition of these groups should be studied at leisure. The focus on detail to build up design is achieved by various methods—sometimes the detail chosen is the wing of an angel, sometimes the pattern is composed by the haloes. A vital figure is dramatised by the scarlet curtain hung behind it, an unimportant one nullified down by a weak position with his face hidden. Note also the pictorial use made of cloaks, swords, staves, water pitchers and baskets in order to strengthen the positions of the important figures. Colour is also used to draw attention to gesture.

Religious plays can carry out all the ideas and even copy exactly the formal grouping of the Heavenly Host, if produced in churches. Careful planning is needed for the grouping, with consideration for the width of the chancel, the height of the altar, the sight lines from the pews and the possibilities of using lighting. Full play can be given to variety in processions, use of different levels, and built-up grouping; but brusque action will strike a jarring note. The platform will often be tiny and congested, which makes it all the more important to employ every possible device to give the effect of movement and change of position. Certain characters should not have to spend long stretches of time marooned on untrustworthy lemonade boxes. All should be planned so that the cast can concentrate entirely on its performance as an act of worship.

In most cases it will be found that a stained glass window attitude is easier to hold than a natural one, and more suitable. Outlines will be largely muffled by robes and draperies, and allowance must be made for this from the first rehearsal. It is disconcerting to take a great deal of trouble over subtle differences of attitude, and find at the dress rehearsal that many of the cast are wrapped in thick grey blankets which must be held on with both hands!

Imaginative use of wings can make a lovely decoration in a dull group. Too often they are crushed together, or make awkward angles, or, until the dress rehearsal, are not considered at all. Cherubs' wings (particularly when viewed from behind) are too touching for words, yet far too often the cherubs are placed facing the audience throughout the play. Angels with long wings and sweeping robes who are posed in profile on steps, should not stand with both feet on the same step—one foot should be on the step above. When sitting on steps, either facing the congregation or in profile, in order to give solidarity to the mass, everyone should sit well back, with erect spines.

Other characters need to be strongly and individually played, but each person must understand the importance of merging into a group and holding an unusual position at certain points in the play.

Religious plays particularly need the stylised pattern. However sincere their religious feeling, a group kneeling with backs to the congregation, showing the soles of its feet with turned-in toes, can be very distracting.

In many religious plays the actors can move quite naturally until the moment the vision appears, or music is heard. Then a group has to hold its position, sometimes while eight verses of a long carol are sung. "Natural" positions held this length of time often look ungainly and unnatural. Very careful grouping and posture is needed if the actor is to freeze into the unobtrusive but important background for the beginning of the heavenly vision. In *Holy Night* there is a moment like this. The characters are a little boy, a street walker, working men and women, etc., who are led by the little boy to the place where he has seen a vision. On their arrival the vision has faded. They are all blaming the boy for taking them away from their drinks, when suddenly he cries out, music is heard and the vision reappears. Now undoubtedly the natural thing for them to do would be to fall on their knees. This takes away the attention from the important point—the vision. In stylised form the group would be arranged in a triangle. If two down-stage and one up-stage, on opposite sides, kneel on the first verse, four on the third verse, three on the fourth verse, none on the fifth and sixth verses, and one reluctantly on the last verse, while the little boy remains standing entranced, the spiritual feeling is heightened.

Positions of prayer can be widely varied; these are divided into three headings—arms, legs, and head.

Legs

1. Standing.
2. Kneeling on one knee.
3. Kneeling on both knees.
4. Sitting back on heels, body erect.
5. Sitting back on heels, body bowed forward.

Head

1. Tilted back, face raised.
2. Erect.
3. Turned to side.
4. Inclined towards shoulder.
5. Dropped forward.

Hands and Arms

1. Arms stretched to full height, palms together, fingers straight.
2. Arms stretched to full height, hands clasped.
3. Elbows bent level with shoulders, palms together, fingers stretched.

4. Elbows bent level with shoulders, hands clasped.

5. Elbows bent level with waist, palms together, fingers stretched.

6. Elbows bent level with waist, hands clasped.

7. Hands crossed on breast.

8. Hands clasped together level with breast.

9. Palms together, fingers straight, level with breast.

10. Hands crossed in front, arms extended downwards.

11. Hands clasped in front, arms extended downwards.

12. Palms together, fingers stretched, arms extended downwards.

It will thus be seen that the highest praying position is a combination of No. 1 position of head and No. 1 position of arms and legs. The lowest kneeling position is the combination of No. 5 legs, No. 5 head, and No. 12 arms position.

A diagonal line of angels kneeling on both knees, with dropped heads, can be heightened by the furthest up-stage kneeling in the same position with raised head.

Two lines meeting in a V up-stage, sitting in position 4, can have their heads all turned towards the other line as if communicating their joy with arms in position 12. This is a good attitude for cherubs at ease. If a sentence has to be pointed they can simultaneously rise to a kneeling position, fold their arms across their chest, and raise their heads to look formal.

For a Nativity group, arrange the cherubs in two semi-circles in front of the crib, which is up-stage centre, half the cherubs facing up-stage, half down, but all heads turned towards the crib, rather as if they were the frame for a picture.

If the right angle is not obtained, an effect very different from the intended one may be made. For instance, an angel had been arranged kneeling on one knee, with both hands reverently clasped on the other knee. When the group was ready he took up his position kneeling, but clasped his elbows and supported himself comfortably on his knee, as one does when waiting for a low catch at cricket. It looked casual and informal to a degree, although the difference in angle was slight. All this means that the actors must know to within an inch where and how they stand. Whether they have hands on their hips, with elbow touching elbow, or elbow going behind the neighbour and touching ribs, or whether alternately elbows make a right angle, makes a tremendous difference to the pattern and the feeling of space and design.

It should not be considered incongruous to arrange a dance for angels. There are occasions on which a producer may feel that more is needed than the usual stately pacing walk, but is at a loss to know how to proceed. Whenever feasible the cherubs should take part as well, as they can more easily be given the sprightly steps. The simplest possible form of pattern and steps should be used. The following dance is meant to be used more as a guide to what is practical than as an example of choreography. Any of the twelve arm positions can be used.

Take eight angels and eight cherubs in whatever pattern is chosen to start the dance, perhaps a circle, and let each cherub stand beside an angel.

ANGELS	CHERUBS
1st Step 8 bars	
Raise both arms to upward spread position. Turn slowly completely round on same spot.	Eight run round angels clockwise. Eight run round angels anticlockwise.
2nd Step 8 bars	
Move forward until each hand touches hand of another angel, forming a smaller circle now, and turn slowly until all are facing outward, arms still raised.	Sit on ground opposite own angel and clap hands in time with music, and on the off beat alternately (4 cherubs on the beat, 4 cherubs off the beat).

3rd Step 8 *bars*

Quick walk on toes, moving round in their circle, right arms raised, left arm crossed on breast.	Still sitting for 1st 4 bars, waving right hand up and down to angels. Rise on 5th bar, run forward and kneel in front of own angel.

4th Step 8 *bars*

Holding both hands of cherub, swing him gently round with quick steps until cherubs are inside angels' circle. Open up into V and run gently into wide V with arms spread, blessing cherubs.	Hold both hands of angel, and swing into centre of angels' circle. Stand still until angels are in position, then *skip* forward and kneel facing own angel.

This dance is usually short enough for such performers to remember easily. They will be able to dance it confidently as the steps are easy, and also to enjoy themselves.

The *Ultra-Modern Play*, written with a religious theme, is usually not suitable to perform in a church. The rather clipped dialogue does not lend itself to church acoustics. These plays usually seem to have a disproportionate number of harlots, and to include feasts, drinking parties, or small, exceptionally informal gatherings which, in one way or another, illustrate decadence. Unless handled discreetly, these scenes can be unpleasant in the extreme, and destroy the whole balance of the play. Outspoken language, combined with sensual movements, which would pass unnoticed in a secular play, can be revoltingly obvious when brought into sharp juxtaposition with religious scenes. While it is clearly the author's intention that these scenes should display the rottenness of vice, it is equally clear that one takes the risk of the audience carrying away in its memory pictures of these scenes as the most outstanding feature of the play.

The safest way of steering between sensationalism and a gentility, that in the circumstances would be ridiculous, is to rely on extremely decorative attitudes and subtle gestures of the head, shoulders, and hands. The seductive body movements suitable for a play like *Hassan* are here entirely out of place and unseemly. It is quite enough for a harlot to walk gracefully, to sit attractively, or recline in a position which shows off her costume; she need not throw herself backwards from the waist, or twine herself around anyone in order to make her status clear. The dialogue in these scenes is usually more than strong enough to convey what is wanted, and does not need underlining visually. Where the scene stipulates an abandoned type of dance, the problem can be tackled in two ways. If the scene is one of orgy, the ultimate effect wanted is probably ugliness, to emphasise the decadence of and corruption of the crowd. Distorted movements, jerking headturns, hunched shoulders, flopping or rigidly stiff fingers, clumsy stamping and exaggerated changes of tempo are all good ingredients for such a scene. Or, one rather grotesque character can be isolated from the group and caper round by himself, occasionally flopping on to the floor or standing still and gazing vacantly. This will point the senseless turmoil of the dancers and the emptiness of their revels.

Masks are often worn in such scenes, and it is very difficult to make the average actor understand how much these really eliminate expression. He will have to work much harder to express his meaning with his whole body. His face will automatically register his feelings, and subconsciously he will feel that that is enough. The producer, in this case, is advised to allow each member in the scene to watch one rehearsal. Until the actor sees for himself how little movement is actually being used, it will be impossible to convince him that the producer is not making unreasonable demands. It may be necessary to rehearse this scene away from the main cast, once at least, if not oftener.

Sometimes Sunday-school children are brought in with

a dance to portray innocent revels, and every effort should be made to see that such a dance is simple as well as decorative. If the dancers are untrained, it is helpful to have long scarves or pieces of material which can be held by two people, one at each end. Pattern can be built up using the contrasting colours of the scarves. This overcomes the greatest difficulty with untrained dancers which is ungraceful arm movement.

It is much easier for them to judge whether the scarf is fully stretched or not, than whether their arms have drooped into ugly angles. The material of the scarf should be flimsy enough to float up and down, but not so lacking in substance that it degenerates into a twisted rag during rehearsals. Poor arm movements can be camouflaged by fluttering gestures, which are easy to make effective by using jingling bracelets. Movements can gain wide variety by maidens choosing flowers out of an enormous basket on the stage. This could help to animate a long passage of dull dialogue. The basket could be placed below the level of the platform, or an imaginary pool could be used. These are useful ways of creating different stage levels. Some of the dancers could stand and some kneel, to look at themselves in the pool. Others could lean forwards, or stand with their backs to the pool, twisting to look over their shoulders at their reflection.

To many Church members, a religious play is the only form of amateur drama that has any value. Certainly the atmosphere at rehearsals can be a revelation to the producer who has not previously tackled such work. The feeling of unselfishness and dedication that such groups generate is extraordinarily moving. It is impressive to the last degree also, to do pioneer work with Youth Groups who have never considered religion and drama as having anything in common, or have possibly never considered religion at all. The growing awareness of the players of being brought into contact with an entirely new element in their lives, and their recognition of how important it is going to be to them, is fascinating to watch. Whether they struggle against it or not, it is impossible for them to ignore it. Producers should beware of how they handle such highly inflammable material, and only approach it, if they are prepared to do so, in a rightly humble way.

CHAPTER X

DANCES IN DRAMA

IN all primitive civilisations and in most advanced ones, dance and drama are inextricably blended; in different forms, tribal and folk dances, ballet, and Greek drama all use dance steps and rhythm to interpret dramatic themes. Dramatised ballads, pageants, and historical plays usually have stylised movements and interpolated dances. These dances have little or no dramatic content, and are merely used as decoration, or to set the period, or in the case of pageants, to use up the folk dances the children have already learnt in class.

For the purposes of historians it is important that dances of a definite period, galliards, pavanes, etc., should be written down and preserved accurately. For stage purposes it is sufficient if an impression of the dance needed is given. One of the reasons for this is obvious: the formations of Court or ballroom dances, intended to be danced on a flat floor for the benefit of the performers, are not theatrically effective. The repetition of steps that enable every lady and gentleman to have a turn in the centre, as in an eightsome reel, are most monotonous to watch. The usual period dance, if carried through correctly, takes too much time away from the play. It is much better to select characteristic steps and formations and present an effect of a minuet or gavotte, than to stick slavishly to historical accuracy.

As a rule the local dancing teacher is called in and, as a rule, this is not to be recommended. Naturally enough, as the dance appears under her name on the programme, she is anxious and competent to make it as good as possible. Unfortunately this means with rare exceptions that the item sticks out immediately as the work of an alien hand instead of contributing to the dramatic atmosphere. The dance is usually rehearsed separately, not enough time is given to explaining to the teacher where the dance fits in or what happens *afterwards*, so that the dance leaves the stage badly prepared for the following scene. It is not suggested that dancing teachers are never to be consulted, they are a mine of information on period and national dances alone, but it is a sound rule that the producer should work out his own dance pattern, rhythm and steps. It is a very moot question if anything is to be gained by the importation of the pupils of a dance school, unless it is clearly stated in the script that professional dancers are intended.

What is essential for the producer, is to fit the *style and steps* peculiar to the dance needed and consider the connection with the costume, which has a marked influence on the movement. The swinging leg of the Charleston, which would catch in the framework of a crinoline, shows off admirably the knee length beaded fringe worn when it was at the height of its vogue. A minuet curtsey will take two bars of 3/4 tempo, which allows full skirts graceful time to sink, swirl, and settle into place again. Done in a short frock, an unpleasing length of time is spent in an awkward bent knee attitude.

Plays containing modern ballroom dancing have many pitfalls. The couples are usually chosen for acting, not dancing, with perhaps two exceptions, who are so startlingly good that the others show up pitifully. In scenes such as the second act of *Johnson over Jordan* or *The Vortex*, characterisation is clearly necessary even in the stereotyped ballroom "hold". These variations are suggested for scenes in which a group is doing modern ballroom dancing in either a night club or a private house.

GIRLS: (A) left arms right round men's necks, (B) both arms round mens' necks, (C) both arms under mens' arms clasping them round waist, (D) both arms under mens' arms, right hands holding men's left shoulders, left hands holding men's right shoulders.

MEN: (A) hold girls' right hands, with elbows bent so both hands are in the middle of girls' backs, (B) both hands held low, one on each side of girls' hips, (C) hold girls' shoulders, fitting their elbows underneath girls' elbows, (D) hands firmly clasped behind girls' backs supporting them as they lean back with arms dangling loosely each side.

It will be seen that in all these positions, contact and control is maintained, and the general effect is of a normal hold. Nothing is suggested that needs a trained dancer. These positions can be tightened up or loosened according to the space and the number of dancers used. They can be done gracefully, merely to achieve variety of pattern, with exaggerated angles and tenseness to suggest abnormality or orgies, or each couple can use all of them in turn to represent a young and virile group exploiting their physical pleasure in the dance. For such scenes the dancers should be most precisely set, so that each couple knows exactly which step it is going to do to get around the corner, and does it every time it rehearses. This particular responsibility need not be the producer's as long as he makes quite certain it is taken over by individuals.

In pageants, to insert folk dances is usually the right procedure, as there are always Kings visiting, and this is one of the accepted ways of entertaining royalty. There is usually no question here as to whether the audience will be bored; if royalty can stand it, so can they. Also the dramatic content of a pageant is necessarily small due to open-air stages and corresponding difficulty in dialogue, so spectacle obviously should take up most of the time.

There is something about a Maypole and dozens of children dancing round it, under a hot sun, with the scent of trampled grass and the sound of the local band, that rightly lulls critical faculties. The audience here will con-

tentedly spend ten minutes watching the children plait
ribbons, while they know very well that they must
presently spend ten minutes watching the same ribbons
being unplaited.

Court dances can be also shown in their entirety as
space is not lacking nor time, and the audience for a
pageant is usually sitting round an arena type of stage and
thus can observe the formation and pattern in a way impossible in an indoor theatre.

Pageants and Chronicle Plays, either out of doors or on
an arena stage, are the place for absolutely accurate
period dances, but if the producer would prefer to use
the theatrical style he could do so.

The most effective *formations for dances* on the stage
are based on simple shapes. Straight lines, circles, stars,
triangles, squares, semi-circles, vary in effectiveness according to the movement used with them.

Straight Lines. Dancers facing each other and moving
backwards and forwards as in "Nuts in May", travelling
side by side down-stage until they part at the footlights
and sweeping round the side of the stage into a semi-
circle, or advancing diagonally across the stage, to split
up into small clusters of three, are all useful for different
purposes.

Circles. These may be varied by having an outer and inner,
either travelling in opposite directions, or one static and
one moving, or mingling as in the Grand Chain in the
Lancers. A small circle down-stage right may be composed
of those actors who have dialogue to put across, contrasted
with a larger circle who only have to dance, placed up-
stage left or spilling over into the centre.

Triangles. These can be used in many different dances, and
are the foundation of most crowd scenes, where certain
characters have odd lines to say which must be clearly
heard.

Semi-Circles. These should be used to focus attention

either on a ceremonial entry or on some important character. They are more effective as a group for they are extremely difficult to keep tidy in a moving formation.

Squares. These need careful thought, as certainly one side of the square will have its back to the audience. Four people make a stingy square. Eight, twelve, or even sixteen are better, and that means that anything up to four backs are steadily displayed to the audience, and those backs block out the four who actually are facing them.

Stars. A stylised form is best used where the points can be emphasised, either by the dancers holding ribbons or garlands or possibly swords or sticks to show the pattern.

The Windmill. Each dancer puts up the right hand towards the centre where all hands meet, and the entire group, facing the same way, moves around in a circle. When arriving back at the same spot, each person turns and offers the left hand to the centre, and the "Windmill" pivots in the opposite direction.

A decorative stage dance should use three or more of these patterns because it is by the patterns, rather than by the steps used, that variety is achieved. The simplest lilting walk or skip, coupled with good carriage of the head and arms, and a suitable type of bow and curtsey, are all that are really needed by any producer for the ordinary dance scene in a play. Patterns are obtained by floor plans and by using alternate performers or groups of performers. If the dance has to work up to a climax the music is quickened, the movements can become loosened or more abandoned but *need not be more complicated or difficult*.

There is very seldom the necessity for any one other than the producer to arrange the dances used, and it is much more satisfactory for everyone concerned if he takes the trouble to do so. It is, incidentally, a welcome change from planning psychological moves, to immerse oneself in a Tarantella.

Two words of command will be needed incessantly,

one is "Stretch" and the other is "Spread out". If the producer sees that something is wrong with the dance but does not quite know what, it is usually either that the dancers are not stretching sufficiently, specially with arms, elbows, and wrists, or else they are huddled together so that the star or circle is not clearly shown.

Period dances invariably commence with the dancers taking up their positions and formations before the music starts and finish in a formal position at the end of the dance. In modern scenes the dancers drift on to the floor, couple by couple, and finish in an equally haphazard manner, stopping at the end of the music, but not always separating or moving off the floor.

If a character is meant to be a ballet dancer, and has, in fact, little or no knowledge of ballet, it is most unwise to allow her to do a pseudo ballet dance to carry out the idea that ballet dancers practise in every spare moment. If it is mentioned in the script that he or she should do so, it is better to keep to an extremely simple movement, such as holding on to a chair with both hands, and raising and lowering the heels. Nothing much can go wrong with this; few things destroy the illusion more than bad ballet arms, and there exists at the moment a very large audience which will instantly recognise inexpert ballet work.

Dances of "allure" are admittedly extremely difficult to arrange, but even here a better effect will be achieved by producer and performer pooling ideas that are within the range of the actress's usual gestures, rather than a teacher imposing definite steps that will preoccupy the actress's mind, and dull the mental projection of her mood. Understanding and choice of music will help more than anything else. Music that is evocative of the mood of the scene, gay, mournful, witty, or nostalgic, is very much more likely to be well chosen by the producer, steeped in the play, than by an outsider responsible for only one part of it.

Folk dances and National dances are more showy if arranged so as to use and to display accessories. If costumes have vivid aprons, handkerchiefs, muffs, they should be arranged accordingly, to use with hand gestures. If swords, staves, or other rigid articles are used, choose a star formation for the beginning and end of the dance. The individual fan or muff can add enormously to the effect of the dance; eight fans simultaneously furling and unfurling will cover a multitude of simple steps.

In both Folk and National dances extra sound effects can be used; clapping hands, stamping feet, shouts of encouragement, eldritch yells as some soloist does his stunt, are all good in different ways. The vocal efforts should not be used until the dance is working up to a climax, clapping is a tidy way of starting everybody at the same moment, and stamping can either be done at the end of a figure, or at the end of the dance. Clapping can heighten the excitement if done by onlookers rather than performers, first one group clapping the rhythm of the music, then another joining in clapping a counter rhythm, until all those not dancing are clapping, and the whole stage is merged into the dance rhythm.

For a funeral dance, wailing or keening can be introduced in this manner, groups starting consecutively until all are swaying and moaning together, and it is difficult to tell who is dancing and who is not.

Sometimes music continues during an entire scene, and pauses can be marked and held longer if, from time to time, a solitary couple can dance for a few minutes and then drift off as the dialogue becomes more important, than if only the music is used.

Finally, a brief *summing up* of the essential quality to bring out in the different types of dance, and some characteristic details:

Folk and National. Vigorous steps, decision in the head movements, strong rhythmic feeling, definite floor pattern.

Period and Court Dances. Dignity and graceful carriage of the head and arms, precise floor pattern, well-rehearsed bows and curtseys, control of costume, swords, etc., curving movements.

Dances of Atmosphere, Allure and Abandonment. No *noticeable* floor pattern, springing steps, and apparently haphazard grouping, free arms, head and body movements.

Ballet. Never to be attempted except by trained ballet dancers.

Symbolic Dances. (Factory workers, rebellions, etc.) Block groups working in straight lines with strong movements, mass effects of simultaneous gestures, very modern music, broken angles, no curves.

Modern Ballroom Dances. Variety of holds, no *noticeable* floor pattern, casual air, desultory start and finish, Quick-Step rather than Slow Fox-Trot or Waltz.

QUESTIONS AND ANSWERS

This chapter deals with a selection of the questions most frequently asked during practical movement sessions, and concerns problems likely to arise for actors, teachers or producers. Perhaps it may be stressed again that everything in this book has been based on personal practical experience extending over many years.

Q. Do you really think the average actor has time for all this "Planned Framework of Movement"? Are you not making it all too complicated?

A. The average actor wastes a great deal of time just because he does not know how to plan a framework. It is far less complicated in the end, and very little more trouble in the beginning, but the most important point is that every bit of work he does is useful afterwards. Otherwise he builds up each separate part piecemeal, and discards the knowledge at the end of the run as inapplicable to another role.

Q. Why should one not use the external approach for children—surely it is much quicker and easier to do with childrens' supple bodies?

A. Because one is aiming at an entirely different target with childrens' drama work. It is *their* imagination that must be stimulated and *their* ideas that must have expression. It is not the object to produce a beautifully finished performance which is merely an echo of the producer's mind.

Q. I would find it impossible to work out a character in in the way you describe. I just know instinctively if a gesture is out of character. Is this wrong?

A. No. Obviously this book is not meant for you, although you might bear two things in mind. What is stated in Chapter II, that a natural gesture is not always theatrically successful, and also the fact that you do it instinctively does not ensure that you would, as a producer, be able to explain to others your reason for doing it.

Q. In our Society we have three dancers who move so beautifully that it looks self-conscious; does not this seem to contradict your theory of trained movement?

A. No. Probably the dancers are self-conscious, certainly if the trained movement is as obvious as all that, the people in question are not in character as regards the play.

Q. I find it very difficult to balance myself correctly, to co-ordinate movement with props, and to gauge distances correctly, so that I do not bump into things. This occupies my mind so much that I cannot really let myself go emotionally. How can I cure it?

A. This difficulty is very often caused by lack of correct focussing of the eyes. Try not to gaze into the audience, and when you are looking at another character, really concentrate your gaze on him, do not just include him in the general area you glance at. It is really a faulty adjustment from the space in real life to the compressed area of the stage.

Q. I have to dance a gavotte with seven others and feel I am very stiff. I have tried everything but cannot cure this. Must I resign my part?

A. You might try remembering that in every age there have been people who found it difficult to dance and never danced well. This mere thought may cause you to relax and forget your stiffness. In the other direction, you might see if you can come to terms between your stiffness and the part you are playing and use pour handicap as part of the characterisation. After all, a gavotte was danced by everyone, it does not need a trained dancer to interpret it competently.

Q. You pay so much attention to what happens when one is actually on the stage; do you not consider it important to get into the mood of the character before one enters?

A. Vitally important, but equally important to display it to the audience once one has entered. One has often seen characters enter in a mood, but what mood was not shown clearly to the audience.

Q. How does one decide in a religious play, where to introduce stylised movement?

A. Usually the cast shows the producer very plainly indeed, where some improvement on the natural position is needed if the religious feeling is not to be hindered from making its effect. The need for music is very often a safe guide as music unco-ordinated with movement is usually rather distracting to the audience.

Q. In Chapter X "Dances in Drama", is there not rather a danger that producers will take the advice too literally about not having Dance Teachers and make ridiculous mistakes?

A. There is always a danger about writing books on practical subjects. This book is intended for intelligent people untrained in this particular subject, and one can only hope that it will help them with their problems and not precipitate them onto other troubles. There is a list of reference books given which should be consulted for accuracy.

Q. We are a scattered group and can only get together for the actual rehearsals. Do you therefore advise practising the exercises separately and alone?

A. Yes, it will always help but what I should rather advise is this. That the punctual arrivers at rehearsals immediately start practising together, and it is made a habit that each newcomer joins in until the entire cast is assembled. This has been tried with great success, the disciplinary value being that the late comers got very little practice. The only drawback is that it finishes up with everyone being so punctual that there is no time for practice.

Q. I was told that all stage gesture was founded on the figure 8. Is this so?

A. In some books on gesture of the eighteenth and nineteenth Century this was an accepted maxim, but it is obviously unsuited to the present form of realistic acting.

Q. I am so conscious of my hands. I have been told "forget them", and try to, but I cannot. What exercises would help?

A. What really helps is knowing that "your" hands are in reality the hands of the character you are portraying. Know what that person would do with them, and the problem of what you do with them need not then arise.

LIST OF REFERENCE BOOKS

DANCES AND ACTING

Elizabethan Dances. NELLIE CHAPLIN. (*Curwen.*)
Orchésographie. ARBEAU. (*C. W. Beaumont.*)
Handbook of European Dance (series). (*MaxParrish.*)
Manners and Movements in Costume Plays. I. CHISMAN and
   H. E. RAVEN HART. (*Deane.*)
Fencing. H. A. COLMAN DUNN. (All England Series 1924.)
   (*G. Bell.*)
Dramatic Art. ENID ROSE. (*University Tutorial Press.*)
The Art of Mime. IRENE MAWER. (*Methuen.*)
The Craft of Comedy. S. HAGGARD and A. SEYLER. (*Muller.*)

DESIGN

English Tradition in Design. J. GLOAG. (*Penguin.*)

MUSIC

Everyman's Dictionary of Music. E. BLOM. (*Dent.*)
Form in Music. S. MCPHERSON. (*Williams.*)
Les Maitres Musiciens de la Renaissance Francaise. (*Augener.*

COSTUME

English Costume of the Early Middle Ages. IRIS BROOKE.
   (*Black.*)
English Costume of the Later Middle Ages. IRIS BROOKE.
   (*Black.*)
English Costume in the Age of Elizabeth. IRIS BROOKE.
   (*Black.*)
English Costume in the 18th Century. IRIS BROOKE. (*Black.*)
English Costume in the 19th Century. IRIS BROOKE. (*Black.*)
Dressing the Part. FAIRFAX PROUDFIT WALKUP. (*Harrap.*)

SUGGESTIONS FOR NATIONAL AND PERIOD DANCES

Middle Ages	Tordion, Pavane, Country Dances, Morris Dances.
16th to 18th Century	Basse Dance, Galliard, Pavane, Bourree d'Achille da Volte.
17th and 18th Centuries	Gavotte, Jig, Minuet, Canaries.
19th Century	Waltz, Polka, Barn Dance, Lancers, Quadrilles, Reels, Galop, Cotillion.
20th Century	Valeta, Tango, Boston Waltz, Charleston, Slow Fox-Trot, Jitterbug.
Russia	Gopak, Trepak.
Germany	Bavarian Schülplatter.
Sicily	Tarantella (snap thumbs or castanets).
Italy	Tarantella (tambourine or castanets).
America	Square Dances.
Denmark	Lime Tree or Maypole Dance.
Bruges	Sword Dance (1389).
Switzerland	Egg Dance (medieval).
Greece	Thessalykos or Cushion Dance.
Portugal	Fish in Basket on head Dance. Flower in Jar on head Dance.
Holland	Groningen Dance.
Finland	Vestvinsk Dance.